M
HANDBOOK

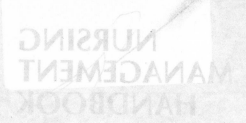

NURSING MANAGEMENT HANDBOOK

Ken Hyett BA MIPM

Principal Lecturer in Management, Brooklands School of Management, Weybridge

Churchill Livingstone

EDINBURGH LONDON MELBOURNE AND NEW YORK 1988

CHURCHILL LIVINGSTONE
Medical Division of Longman Group UK Limited

Distributed in the United States of America by Churchill
Livingstone Inc., 1560 Broadway, New York, N.Y. 10036,
and by associated companies, branches and
representatives throughout the world.

First published 1988

ISBN 0-443-03626-8

British Library Cataloguing in Publication Data
Hyett, Ken
   Nursing management handbook.
   1. Management   2. Nursing service
   administration
   I. Title
   658'.0024613   RT89

Library of Congress Cataloging in Publication Data
Hyett, Ken.
   Nursing management handbook.
   Includes bibliographies and index.
   1. Nursing services — Administration.   2. Health
services administration.   3. National Health Service
(Great Britain)   I. Title.   [DNLM: 1. Nursing,
Supervisory — handbooks. WY 39 H9955]
   RT89.H94   1988   362.1'73'068   87-14695

Produced by Longman Singapore Publishers (Pte) Ltd.
Printed in Singapore

Preface

The decision to make a career in nursing is usually taken from a general desire to help others. Often the individual will only have a limited understanding of the real interests, rewards and problems that are likely to be found in the profession. Similarly, in other occupations career choices are made from rather generalised impressions of what it is like to be a civil engineer, a school teacher, a social worker or computer scientist. It can be ironic, therefore, to find after several years training and success as a practitioner in a chosen profession, that promotion to a more senior appointment can impose such radical changes in the nature of work that it is almost like starting in a new career.

A teacher taking up a headship for the first time will no longer be required to practise the basic craft of classroom teaching. The more senior the post in engineering the less involvement there will be with practical engineering tasks. A similar experience is likely to occur to those promoted through the ranks of nursing and other health care professions. A nurse who selected this career from an interest and enthusiasm for the tasks of directly caring for patients and who has actually found satisfaction from this, will find a steady reduction in the amount of time to be spent in patient care on promotion to charge nurse/ward sister. This is accentuated with further promotion through the senior nurse grades to director of nursing services or a post

as general manager. Time will be spent away from the hospital ward or community setting completing administrative paperwork, reading budget summaries, organising training, running meetings etc. When this happens a nurse has really entered a new profession requiring acquisition of the additional knowledge and skills of nurse management. Such a transition is inevitable, but the reality of this change is not always expected or welcomed.

Some senior nurses talk rather regretfully about the decline in patient contact or find it difficult to be enthusiastic about the administrative aspects of their work. However, such attitudes are not universal. It is encouraging that many senior nurses do find promotion brings rewards from the acceptance of greater responsibility and meeting fresh challenges. There is an opportunity to influence the overall standards of nursing care in a section, to contribute to the development of nursing staff and to be a respected member of a management team.

Many nurses, however, are sceptical about the relevance of management techniques to the needs of health care. They associate 'management' with a lack of concern for patient needs, with an emphasis on costs or cutting back on service. Nurses should be cautious about the application of concepts that have been developed in the world of business. Health care is unique and requires a particular style of management. However, an important characteristic of the nursing profession is a willingness to seek new ideas by learning and research.

The aim of this book is to describe various theories and practices of management in general and then to consider how these can be applied by senior nurses. There is a deliberate attempt to present general concepts first and to compare the problems of managing a nursing service with those of managing other organisations. Whilst we acknowledge the unique circumstances of nurse management, the purpose here is to encourage nurses to think like managers when dealing with the practical problems of running a hospital ward or a community service.

It is hoped that the book will be useful to those already holding a nurse management post by encouraging them to review their present approach to managing and adding to their knowledge of management techniques. For readers hoping to be promoted, or just taking up a more senior appointment, the book should be useful in developing a wider understanding of management skills that are relevant to making a success of a new managerial post.

The book is divided into four sections. The first examines the general question of what is involved in being a good manager before looking at the specific issue of managerial effectiveness and nursing. The second section also gives a broad introduction to organisational theories before describing organisational structures of the National Health Service. The third section contains the main theme of the book as it describes a variety of general management skills and considers how these could be used by nurse managers. The final section describes some broader management techniques that are used in running health care organisations.

The book can either be read as a whole in the order presented, or specific parts can be studied by nurses looking for information on particular aspects of management. In order that sections can be read separately there is reference to other parts of the book and a limited amount of repetition. This is not intended as an academic study of the problems involved in managing health care services but as a practical handbook to help nurse managers deal with problems involved in running a section of the nursing service. The techniques described and the recommendations concerning their application by managers are based on well-accepted theories and practice. References to particular authorities and research studies have, however, been generally avoided in the text. At the end of each chapter there are lists of suggested further reading and references on which the content has been based. I have also drawn on my personal experience as a manager and management trainer. This has involved me with many managers and organisations from industry and commerce as well as extensively with those from the NHS and the independent health sector. In researching this particular book I consulted with many nurse managers from ward level upwards. The aim of the book remains that of looking outside the confines of nursing for skills and techniques of management which can be applied successfully by senior nurses. This seems to be particularly relevant for nurses, given the developments in management of the 1980s in the NHS as well as in private medicine.

Throughout the book the term 'she' has been used in reference to individual nurse managers although the content applies equally to men and women managers.

K.H.   Weybridge, 1988

Contents

SECTION FOUR	**Management techniques and health care**	

SECTION ONE

Managerial effectiveness

1

An introduction to management

WHAT IS MANAGEMENT?

In trying to answer the apparently simple question, 'What is management?'it is necessary to consider the differences between the various jobs that exist in most work places. Whether we look at a large general hospital, a nursing home, a major bank, a supermarket chain or a construction company it is possible to identify five distinct categories of job:

— The direct workforce
— The indirect workforce
— The supervisory staff
— The middle management
— The senior management.

The direct workforce

The first obvious group of jobs includes those concerned with carrying out the tasks that are essential for the actual production of an organisation's goods or services. This group can be called collectively the direct workforce. Thus cashiers in banks are directly involved with providing the tangible services offered to customers; assembly workers in a manufacturing company directly contribute to the final products that are sold to customers, and engineers in an electronics company spend their time making products.

The indirect workforce

In all but the smallest organisations there will

be a second group of workers who are engaged in clerical work to provide the administration and information systems that are required for the efficient operation of a business or public service. Others will be engaged in manual and technical work needed to maintain the assets and resources of the organisation (buildings, machinery, equipment etc.). These jobs can be regarded as part of the indirect workforce as they are not primarily concerned with providing services or goods for the 'customers' of an organisation.

Supervisory staff

A third distinct group of jobs includes those responsible for ensuring that the efforts of a particular section of the direct or indirect workforce are individually effective and properly co-ordinated. Individuals in these posts are the first line of management (usually called supervisory management). Some may be engaged in clerical, professional or manual work similar to that of their work group, but their main responsibility will be to ensure that this section works effectively. In many cases the job titles will not include the work manager or supervisor. Instead, other titles indicating supervisory responsibility will be used such as: section head, leading hand, senior clerk, chargehand, team leader etc.

Middle management

A fourth group of jobs that exist in larger organisations incorporates those with responsibility for the supervision of supervisors and the control of larger sections of the workforce, direct or indirect. The term middle management is often applied to such jobs, as they are the link between the first line management and the most senior management.

Senior management

The fifth distinct category is made up of those jobs with responsibility for developing the overall policy and objectives of a whole organisation or business enterprise and the systems

and procedures that are needed to achieve these corporate aims. This is the senior management. In commercial organisations they may be directors and members of the company board. Similarly in public service organisations there will be senior posts with the title of director involving membership of a senior management committee.

Line and staff managers

In all organisations, management will be made up of junior, middle and top managers. Thus a workshop foreman in a factory should be as much 'management' as the works director or the chief accountant. It is usual to make some further distinctions within management posts, however, between those regarded as 'line' management and those variously called 'staff, functional or specialist' management.

Line managers can be located at junior, middle or senior levels in a hierarchy. The distinctive feature of such posts is that they are responsible for running sections or larger units that contain the direct workforce. They are the managers charged directly with producing a satisfactory quality and quantity of goods or services to the organisation's customers.

Staff or functional specialists can also be located at any place in the hierarchy. At the lower levels they are responsible for ensuring proper support is given to line departments so that they can function properly. At the senior levels they are responsible for advising senior line management and general managers on the appropriate organisational policies in their particular specialisms. Common functional areas are those in personnel and training, research and development, marketing and advertising, public relations, supplies, management services etc.

There is an essential role in all organisations that ensures that the line and functional specialists work together for the final purpose of achieving organisational aims. This responsibility is usually vested ultimately in the post of managing director, chief executive at the top of an organisation or of regional general manager or plant manager at a lower level.

THE MANAGING PROCESS

There have been many attempts to produce a universally applicable description of this process of managing. One of the most frequently quoted descriptions is:

to manage is to forecast and to plan, to organise, to command, to co-ordinate and to control.
(Fayol 1967)

Other well known references on the same topic are:

Executive work is not that of the organisation, but the specialised work of maintaining the organisation in operation.
(Renold 1949)

Management is the process of getting things done through the agency of a community.
(Barnard 1958)

One can define the work of the manager as planning, organising, integrating and measuring.
(Grove 1983)

Such definitions can appear to be over-authoritarian ('command', 'getting things done') and rather too generalised to be of great practical use.

A more detailed analysis of the management process would break it down into five major activities.

Establishing objectives

It is necessary in organising any type of work to have a clear view of the main purpose or target to be achieved. Then priorities and standards can be identified and eventually an assessment of results can be made.

Planning and organising

From an identification of objectives it is necessary to make plans which indicate the resources required (people, materials, equipment, systems, finance) and how these can be put together to obtain the desired results.

Influencing and motivating

The actual work of an organisation is not carried out by managers. Managers are essentially concerned with ensuring that workers are competent, committed and co-operative enough to achieve the desired results.

Monitoring and controlling

It is essential to include in plans the means of getting information about progress and whether standards have been maintained. It is also necessary to ensure proper co-ordination and speedy decision-making to adjust to changing conditions.

Reviewing and developing

The demands of an organisation are constantly changing as there are fluctuations in the community or market it serves. It is essential to review and to measure the extent to which objectives are being met, as well as whether the objectives themselves are still appropriate. It is necessary to examine the quality of organisational systems, structures, policies and staff so that these can be developed to meet the demands of the future.

Management in practice does not appear as such a logical and systematic process. Most organisations have ambiguities, anomalies, apparent waste and contradictions. Yet if efficiency and quality are to be achieved, it is necessary that this managerial cycle is practised at corporate level and in the various subsections. Thus managing is an activity which is carried out by everyone who holds a post of responsibility, with discretion in their work which requires planning, monitoring, influencing and reviewing.

. . . . the first criterion in identifying those people within an organisation who have management responsibility is not command over people. It is responsibility for contribution.
(Drucker 1968)

EFFECTIVE MANAGERS

It can be difficult for first-line supervisors and for senior professional or technical staff to identify their management role. Team leaders, section heads and advisors only spend part of

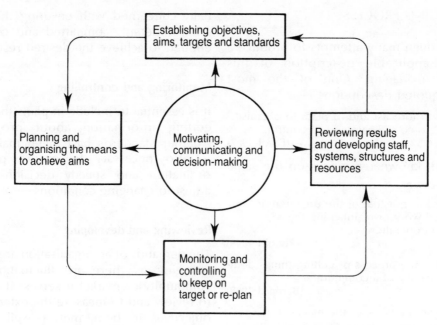

Fig. 1.1 The management process. This process applies to complete organisations as well as to the management of specific sections, projects and individual tasks.

their time planning, organising etc., the remainder of their time being devoted to carrying out similar tasks to their team, or actually producing goods or providing services personally.

A common problem for working supervisors or professional team leaders is to decide the appropriate balance between 'operational' tasks and those of administration and managing. Clearly the first priority should be given to managing. This is essential to enable a group of staff to work efficiently or to ensure one's own work is properly organised. Unfortunately, pressures are such that many find they are too busy 'working' to give time to planning and monitoring.

Each supervisory post has different press-ures demanding that a particular balance of time should be devoted to managerial and operational tasks in order to achieve satisfac-tory results. An essential question for all managers is: 'Have I got the balance right?'

There are many factors involved in becoming an effective manager and many views on how to achieve managerial success.

Most established managers have their own formula drawn from their own experiences. There have been many attempts to find a generally applicable prescription, ranging from a massive research study of 2 000 managers in 500 top US industrial companies which identified 18 key managerial competences (Lillebo, 1982) (see Fig. 1.2) to more simple recommendations in popular books such as the *One Minute Manager* (Blan-chard & Johnson 1983) with one minute goal setting, one minute praisings and one minute reprimands. Depending on your source of guidance, a manager can be variously advised to communicate effectively, to exercise firm control by detailed planning, to have influ-ence with higher management, to be positive, to be innovative, to control use of time etc. The problem with taking such apparently useful advice is that it tends to concentrate on the means of managing rather than the results.

The only generally acceptable definition of an effective manager is the most obvious — one who achieves the required results. These

This study of 2000 managers identified a number of common skills requirements for effective managers irrespective of the type of organisation involved. These are:

Intellectual	Logical thought
	Conceptualisation
	Diagnostic use of concepts
Entrepreneurial	Effective use of available resources
	Taking initiatives
Socio-emotional	Self-control
	Spontaneity
	Perceptual objectivity
	Stamina and adaptability
Interpersonal	Self-confidence
	Developing others
	Impact and influence
	Use of unilateral power
	Use of socialised power
	Oral communication
	Positive regard of others
	Managing group processes

Fig. 1.2 Competences of management success (American Management Association 1982).

may be measured by the quantity and quality of output from a work group against costs incurred, or, in the case of specialist support staff, assessed by such factors as numbers of staff recruited, training days organised, projects completed or new systems implemented.

An effective manager is one who is able to select the means, the techniques and the approaches that are most likely to achieve the results required, rather than one who always employs the same formula, either from a belief that it is correct management or from ignorance of an alternative. This does not imply that the end justifies the means. Clearly, managers have social and human responsibilities: the means and the ends should reflect these. In general it is best to communicate regularly with staff, to be considerate of their needs, to praise, to try to develop co-operative relations and to be innovative. However, there are circumstances when it is appropriate to be more distant, more directive or where confrontation and disruption can be the best strategy. To be an effective 'results

oriented' manager it is useful to observe nine key points:

1. To be clear on the results expected in your particular role — what are the objectives, goals, standards, targets? Can these be expressed in tangible and measurable terms?
2. To develop this understanding of objectives from constructive discussion with your immediate senior managers and others dependent on the work output of your unit
3. To share this understanding of objectives and demands with your own staff if you are a team leader
4. To ensure that subordinate staff in turn have a clear view of what is expected of them, together with the skills and resources to achieve this
5. To have an understanding of the options available in planning and organising work to meet the goals
6. To have reliable information available indicating the extent to which work is progressing on target
7. To make appropriate and final decisions in the light of reliable information
8. To review personal and subordinate effectiveness fairly and regularly
9. To learn from experience and to be open-minded in approach to management and to people

These points may be regarded as obvious and only the application of common sense. Of course they are, but in my experience in diagnosing management training needs and conducting management training in many different organisations, I have found that these basic principles of good management are often ignored. The most fundamental need is for clarity of purpose.

Many businesses try to ensure that all managers are clear about objectives and that these link together to underpin corporate goals. A formal system called 'Management by Objectives' (MBO) found considerable favour in the 1970s. This requires top management to specify the overall aims and specific objectives that a business is to achieve. In turn there should be discussions between the managers and their subordinate managers to clarify individual responsibilities and the most important aspects of each unit and job ('Effectiveness areas' or 'Key result areas') so that tangible and qualified objectives are agreed for each individual, which contribute to the overall corporate objectives. These individual goals are recorded and form the basis of regular review meetings between subordinates and their immediate managers throughout the organisation.

It is clear that an official and integrated MBO scheme requires considerable investment in time to clarify roles, and to review targets. It also needs accurate information to be provided to managers so that they can monitor progress. In this ultimate form MBO can be over-mechanistic and need substantial administration, which can become counterproductive. Thus the system has rather fallen from favour although the underlying principles are central to effective management.

There is another dilemma for management trying to make precise definitions of targets and standards, which is that individual middle managers and supervisors may feel that these have been imposed on them and are unrealistic; yet it is essential to have clarity of purpose.

Managers should aim to develop mutual agreement on general priorities of roles and interpretation of these into more specific objectives. Imposing targets on others without their commitment will only lead to defensive and restrictive responses.

The principles which should apply in establishing objectives are that they should be:

Equitable — Everyone in a unit is working to equally demanding standards.
Essential — Targets are seen as of significance to some desirable goal.
Attainable— Individuals will have sufficient flexibility, authority, scope and resources to have a reasonable chance of meeting the targets.
Adjustable— If individuals perform well but targets are unattainable some adjustment will be possible.
Inviolable — Meeting targets will not simply result in targets being tightened.

You may consider that such a results-oriented view of manager effectiveness is applicable to businesses manufacturing goods to be sold in the market place for a profit, but is not relevant to services developed for humanitarian ends. Agreed, it is easier to identify specific and measurable goals for production departments in manufacturing cars, microprocessors or television receivers. But we all work in organisations with limited financial resources and are all required to justify the use of these resources through benefits provided. Although it may be difficult to measure the quality of educational output of a middle school, or the value of research undertaken by a research institute, as well as being philosophically unpleasant to ask a charitable organisation to exercise financial restraint, these are the inescapable tasks of all people who accept posts of responsibility.

This does not mean that health care managers should adhere blindly to a concept of ruthless management that might be necessary for survival in some highly competitive commercial enterprises. Managers have to work out the appropriate means for achieving the end of satisfactory health care within the constraints imposed in working for a public service with public accountability.

From this general review of the main content of managing and the concept of managerial effectiveness we shall consider their application to the particular setting of nursing and managing nursing services.

REFERENCES

Barnard C 1958 The functions of an executive. Oxford University Press Oxford

Blanchard K, Johnson S 1983 The one minute manager Fontana, Glasgow.

Drucker P 1968 The practice of management. Pan Books, London

Fayol H 1967 General and industrial management Pitman, London

Grove A 1983 High output management. Souvenir Press, London

Lillebo A 1982 Profile 26, American Management Association

Renold Sir C The nature of management, British Institute of Management, Occasional Paper Number 2

2

Effective nurse management

It is possible to identify four main require-ments which every nurse manager must meet in seeking to be fully competent. First it is essential to understand what results are expected in a particular role, then it is necessary to allocate time and energy in a way that is appropriate to achieving these results. On top of this it is important to have the skills and knowledge needed to carry out these activities. Then it is necessary to get information which can indicate whether results are forthcoming and to decide how future improvements could be made.

In starting with a clear view of aims and priorities for a particular role and a particular part of a nursing service it is necessary to add a broader appreciation of the overall aims and priorities of health care today.

SETTING STANDARDS

In the case of the National Health Service, overall aims are established between the Government via the DHSS and the Health Service Supervisory Board (see Ch. 3 for fuller account). Broadly the intention is to deliver health care equally to the whole population, whilst meeting the special needs of local communities and staying within the agreed financial allocations. The exact interpretation of these aims into specific objectives, whether in fact these are realistic aims at all, has been, and will continue to be, the subject of considerable debate. It is outside the scope of this book to examine the issues involved in setting the appropriate role for public medicine in our society. There are many publications dealing with this topic in great depth. We shall consider the means by which individual nurse managers can establish results and standards for a specific role and how assessments of effectiveness can then be made.

There are several sources of guidance for individual job holders. One is the official job description. This should give details of responsibilities, tasks, reporting and supervisory relationships, as well as the job title and overall objectives or 'key results areas'.

If we examine two examples of nurse manager job descriptions, this will illustrate the problems and possibilities of establishing practical job objectives from this source.

One is a senior nurse in operating and recovery wards, the other a clinical nurse manager, night duty. Both have statements of overall purpose.

Senior clinical nurse: job summary:

The Senior Clinical Nurse, under the direction of the Principal Nurse, is accountable for overall administration of the Operating Departments and Recovery Wards. He/She will be responsible for achieving and maintaining acceptable standards of nursing care, theatre practice and management, and training of learners.

Clinical nurse manager, night duty: job summary:

1. Participating in managing and controlling the night nurse services, with specific responsibility for the Orthopaedic Unit. Acting as professional advisor on all matters concerning patient care within the unit.
2. Identifying the learning needs of the learners and qualified staff, acting as an educator and facilitator for all staff on night duty.

In these descriptions the key results areas are expressed in rather broad terms, 'maintaining appropriate nursing standards', 'identifying learning needs'. The actual definition of nursing standards has to be evolved from discussion and negotiation with the senior line manager, taking into account individual

intention, staffing and other resources available. This is likely to present some problems, in all nurse management appointments.

For example, Ward Sister in a unit dealing with disturbed geriatric patients will have clear views from her professional commitment on what constitutes 'appropriate standards', part of which will include an assessment of patient abilities on entry and active care to maintain these. The staff — patient ratio allocated may not allow time for such detailed assessment and individual care. Thus the prevailing view of an appropriate standard of nursing care will have to be based on compromise between ideal professional aims and the particular resources available. Thus there are likely to be two sets of objectives. One is the set introduced by a manager from her perceptions, experiences and ambitions. The other is the set imposed from more senior managers reflecting the constraints and aims of the whole organisation. In some circumstances the manager will want to set higher standards of achievement and provision of services than the organisational aims require. In other circumstances the individual will wish to have lower targets than those set by higher levels of management.

In addition to the problem of conflicting interpretation of aims there is the usual difficulty that the detailed tasks set for a nurse manager are not capable of exact definition, or precise measurement. In the two senior nurse posts referred to above many of the detailed areas of responsibility need more exact definition if results are to be expressed in measurable terms:

'initiating and developing new methods and ideas'

'ensuring that night nursing care is maintained at the highest level'

'exercising effective leadership to ensure clear staff relationships, good morale'.

Again agreement must be reached by interpretation between the senior nurse and the director of nursing services as well as with ward sisters reporting to the senior nurse.

We have seen the difficulties that are likely to be encountered in writing precise objectives for nurse managers; it will also be apparent from the examination of job descriptions that there may be other anomalies that have to be clarified. One of the senior nurse posts refers to the job holder as being 'Accountable to the Director of Nursing Services' whilst also 'Reporting to the Assistant Director of Nursing Services'.

It is essential to establish a practical interpretation of such situations, otherwise the senior nurse is in danger of facing the stress of having two bosses who do not necessarily share the same view about reporting and accountability.

Although precise standards of nursing performance may be difficult to establish, there are several other possible sources of definition. One set emerges from ward procedure manuals, written standard nursing orders and ward plans. A second set emerges from agreement with doctors and other members of a health care team on desired nursing provision for the particular specialism and individual patients, which are reflected in individual nursing care plans. Above this are the codes of conduct inherent in the professional training of nurses and medical staff.

In recent years there have been attempts to establish additional standards as 'indicators of performance' to judge the efficiency of a unit or hospital. Such factors as comparative length of stay for inpatients with particular conditions, the level of bed occupancy, costs per outpatient day, length of waiting lists, have been given a national standard against which particular units can be measured or which can be used to set management targets. The system of budgetary control sets precise financial standards for each unit and gives the budget holder a further definition of aims and results. Exercise one contains a simple activity which can be used in the first stage of reviewing managerial effectiveness. It is intended to help individuals consider the objectives, standards and results that are applicable in a post.

With a clear agreement on what is expected from a job between those in higher authority and the individual job holder it is possible to consider whether an individual is effective. This involves the primary question, 'How far are the results achieved satisfactory?' If the end product is judged acceptable a senior nurse could, with justification, claim to be an effective manager. There are some supplementary questions to be answered before this judgement is accepted completely: 'Could better results have been achieved?', 'Could the same results have been achieved with less effort or fewer difficulties?' 'Will circumstances change in the future?' Answers to these questions can suggest that changes in approach by a senior nurse could be helpful, or that some improvements in knowledge and skill are required. The problem remains of where this improvement should be made.

ASSESSING PERFORMANCE

Although each nurse management post has precise responsibilities, it is possible to identify five main elements common to nurse line managers. These are managerial tasks, administrative tasks, direct teaching, professional development activities and direct clinical work (see Fig. 2.1). Thus the first consideration in case of doubt on an individual's management performance is whether the proper amount of time and energy is devoted to the management aspect. Some newly appointed staff are reluctant to relinquish clinical work; others spend too much time at their desk on administration.

The first priority for ward sisters/charge nurses is to ensure that nursing staff are available, are properly equipped and resourced, and are sufficiently capable, informed and motivated to provide the necessary standard of nursing care. This involves management. Thus it can be argued that direct clinical work is the lowest priority behind teaching, professional development and administration. At more senior levels of nurse line management there is a similar breakdown of major tasks with similar priorities, but probably little or no direct nursing.

1. Management tasks	Agreeing objectives, planning, organising work, monitoring work, controlling work, liaison, communication, motivating, reviewing and developing
2. Administrative tasks	Clerical activities which are required to keep a unit/ward functioning but do not require managerial decisions
3. Direct teaching	Teaching juniors is part of the management task of developing staff, but distinction can be made between assessing training needs, planning programmes and actually teaching personally
4. Professional development activities	Senior nurses are employed to provide up-to-date advice on particular aspects of nursing care. It is necessary to undertake personal study and research to update knowledge and skills
5. Direct clinical work	Senior nurses are required to advise nurses on clinical practice and to make contact with patients. This is part of the management activity but distinction should be made between these tasks and that of personally providing patient care

Fig. 2.1   The main elements of effectiveness for nurse managers.

Exercise 1 Assess your effectiveness as a nurse manager

1. List the 'key result areas' of your present job and indicate the standard of result you need to achieve in each.

Key result areas   Standards

2. How far have you reached the required standard in each of the key areas above?

Key area   Results obtained

	Excellent always	Generally good	Could be better	Very poor

3. Specify the main patient care objectives of the unit/ward/service for which you are responsible.

4. How do you rate the results obtained by your unit/ward/service in terms of direct patient care or in contribution to patient care? (Example indications)

	Excellent	Good	Poor	Very poor
a. Patient comfort				
b. Patient amenities				
c. Spending against budget				
d. Cost control				
e. Bed occupancy				
f.				
g.				
h.				
i.				

In advisory and functional posts, nurses will have management and administrative tasks together with a need for professional development activities. The teaching tasks can be replaced, or augmented, by direct advising and informing of staff. Direct clinical tasks may be replaced or augmented by direct technical or other practical work in a particular field of expertise.

Exercise Two requires some analysis of the way priorities are determined between these main aspects of nurse management.

Although we are concerned with managerial competence, clearly each element affects the others. If a ward sister lacks knowledge of a hospital administrative system, or is not skilled in controlling her paperwork, the administration tasks will take more time and energy than they should. To improve her effectiveness as a manager she may first need to speed up the processing of administrative chores. Similarly, if a ward sister lacks confidence in her teaching ability she may either do less than she should or find that the energy required distracts her from other tasks.

Thus the key to management effectiveness is self-assessment and self-development. These processes cannot be carried out in isolation, however. It is necessary to understand how others assess your performance.

In the case of a ward sister, it will be necessary to take account of the views of several others. Doctors with patients in a ward will have opinions based on their perceptions of the role of nurses. Nursing staff will have views about the way a ward sister provides clinical leadership, about her teaching input and about her managerial style. Heads of ancillary services and ancillary workers themselves will also make judgements. Patients will have strong views about the quality of nursing care they receive, thus providing the ultimate judgement of the overall performance of a nurse manager.

You may regard the suggestion of trying to understand how others rate your job performance, especially more junior staff or those in other professions, as at best laughably impractical or at worst downright dangerous. If you are a committed professional and appreciate that the delivery of good health care is a team activity, the concept of and mutual appraisal will not seem so far-fetched or threatening.

In trying to make an honest estimate of how others see you it is likely that many readers will have to record 'no idea' in some sections. It is possible to work with someone for many years and yet have no direct indication from them on how they regard you as a subordinate or colleague. Indeed, a common complaint amongst more junior staff is that seniors are usually willing to point out when things go wrong, yet rarely give praise when everything goes smoothly, and never give overall constructive feedback of performance.

Exercise 2 Allocation of priorities

1. What proportion of your time or energy *should* you give to the five elements of your job? (see Fig. 2.1)

	Time %	Energy %
Management tasks		
Administration tasks		
Direct teaching/advising		
Professional development		
Direct clinical/technical/ professional work		
Others		

2. Try to recall at the end of each shift/day how you used your time and energy.

	Management %	Administration %	Direct teaching %	Professional dev. %	Direct clinical %	Other %
Day 1						
2						
3						
4						
5						

3. How does the picture in question 2 compare with your views in question 1?

Exactly the same	Broadly the same	Rather different	Very different

4. How satisfied are you with the way you allocate your time and energy between these main tasks?

Very
satisfied

Generally
satisfied

Some change
needed

Considerable
change needed

5. How could you improve the balance of your time/energy allocation?

Examples:

a. Do you spend too much time on direct clinical activities at the expense of administration?

b. Do you spend too much time on routine administration tasks at the expense of coaching nursing staff, influencing senior nurses etc?

c. Do you spend too much time on direct teaching of learners at the expense of advising and supporting experienced staff?

d. Do you spend too much time advising on patient care at the expense of administration?

e. Do you spend too much time at meetings away from the ward/unit at the expense of monitoring ward staff?

f. Do you spend too much time on administration at the expense of professional development?

After consideration of the correct priorities that should be attached to a particular post the next step in assessing effectiveness is to evaluate the existing level of knowledge and skill for each main component. This is included in Exercise three.

Exercise 3 Personal effectiveness

---

1. Management tasks
How do you rate your current effectiveness in the main management activities listed below?

a. Establishing objectives for self and staff
   (i) Self

Completely clear on my objective	Generally clear on my objective	Rather vague on my objective	No clear objective

   (ii) Staff

All my staff have clear objectives	Most staff generally clear on objectives	Most staff vague about objectives	No clear objective

b. Planning and organising

I am totally effective	Generally effective	Could be better	Very poor

c. Monitoring and controlling

Fully in control of section work	Generally in control	Could be more in control	Serious lack of control

d. Influencing and motivating others
   Assess the quality of your relationship with various individuals on the scale:

Fully able to influence/ motivate	Generally able to influence/ motivate	Could be better at influencing/ motivating	Very poor at influencing/ motivating

   (i) Immediate senior nurses

   (ii) Own staff

    (iii) Nurse management
         colleagues

    (iv) Doctors

    (v) General manager

    (vi) Others

e. Reviewing and developing

Frequent review with staff and making development plans	Some reviews and development plans	Should have more reviews and development plans	No reviews, no development

2. Administration tasks

How do you rate your performance in carrying out routine administration and supervising administrative routines? Excellent   Generally good   Could be better   Very poor

a. Knowledge of administration systems

b. Accuracy and speed of work

3. Teaching task
How do you rate your current performance in teaching learners in your ward/unit?

- a. Content of teaching
  Excellent　　　　Generally good　　　　Could be better　　　　Very poor

- b. Planning and preparation
  Excellent　　　　Generally good　　　　Could be better　　　　Very poor

- c. Delivery
  Excellent　　　　Generally good　　　　Could be better　　　　Very poor

4. Professional development tasks
How do you rate your performance in increasing your knowledge and skills in relevant clinical/technical aspects?
Excellent　　　　Generally good　　　　Could be better　　　　Very poor

What are the clinical/technical aspects you should develop?

5. Clinical tasks
How would you rate your skills as a practical nurse in the specialism of your ward/unit.
Excellent　　　　Generally good　　　　Could be better　　　　Very poor

Although it is much easier to work for a senior who does provide proper feedback or to be part of an official appraisal system, it is still possible for an individual manager to initiate conversations when formal feedback has been missing. The easiest will be with your own immediate team of staff and supervisors. Indeed such activities are implied in the job description of many senior nurses: 'Identify training needs'; 'Develop attitudes and awareness'; 'Carry out appraisals and performance reviews'. The purpose of meetings within a unit team should be to engage in open and mutual review of performance, looking at good points and agreeing on aspects for improvement. Thus a ward sister should try to get views from staff nurses on her contribution to the unit effectiveness as well as giving her view of the nurses' effectiveness.

Another widely available source of information for assessing your own effectiveness is from talking with colleagues in a similar role, either in the same hospital or elsewhere. Comparisons of organisational arrangements, priorities, resources and problems can suggest how well or otherwise you are doing, as well as giving some useful practical ideas for improvement.

It is more difficult, but certainly not impossible, to arrange a meeting with someone higher in the organisation with a view to getting information on your strengths and weaknesses. If this does seem too difficult or threatening in the absence of an official appraisal scheme, it might still be feasible to develop informal conversations to draw out comments from seniors on how they regard your effectiveness. In a similar way it will be useful to arrange periodic review meetings with heads of other sections like domestic services.

Probably the most difficult relationship to review in such an open way is that involving medical staff. Acknowledged by many ward sisters and senior nurses as at least an ambiguous feature, if not the most trying aspect, of their managerial responsibility, it is still essential to have a constructive review of effectiveness with the relevant doctors.

A common outcome of getting a greater insight into how various people rate your effectiveness is that there will be conflicting opinions. A senior nurse might regard a ward sister as too weak in controlling nursing staff, whilst the staff may consider her to be too aloof and dictatorial. This is an occupational hazard for all managers. Professional survival rests on being able to achieve a reasonable balance between conflicting demands.

A näive view of a bureaucratic organisation would suggest that the views of an immediate superior are the most authoritative, as staff in more senior posts are supposed to have greater experience, knowledge and skill than those in more junior posts. In reality this is not always the situation. Whilst not agreeing with the view which suggests that senior posts have been filled by people who have reached their level of incompetence, it does have some observable confirmation. This is particularly so in organisations employing professional specialists in junior positions, as the problem of professional and technical obsolescence will affect many older senior staff.

Indeed, in talking to hundreds of managers in different organisations I have found few who hold their immediate bosses in high esteem. Ironically, I have found that most managers believe that their own staff have a high regard for them. Problems over co-operation are regarded as the fault of the subordinate rather than that of the manager himself. We consider this phenomenon in more detail in Chapter 13.

IMPROVING EFFECTIVENESS

There is no absolutely reliable and completely objective means of assessing managerial competence. A nurse manager has to consider available information on her performance in the managerial, teaching, administrative, professional development and clinical aspects of a particular role. Some will be relatively factual, such as expenditures against budget, treatments completed, bed occupancy, patient assessments made or teaching sessions conducted. Others will be, as we have seen, subjective and possibly conflicting opinions of staff, seniors and colleagues. Ultimately, every nurse manager has to take account of all these indicators, as well as the general standards and trends emerging from the nursing and health care professions, to make some overall self-assessment of present effectiveness. From such a review, a nurse manager should be able to identify particular objectives for improving present performance and, if appropriate, for improving chances of promotion to a higher grade post. Once targets have been specified, then practical plans can be made to achieve these, and after a suitable period further assessment made of the level of actual attainment (see Ch. 19).

Thus the ultimate measure of effectiveness in nurse management, as in any other responsible post in every organisation, is the willingness of an individual to accept the responsibility for self-development. This requires an open-minded outlook; willingness to seek criticism and praise from others; desire to learn from experiences and from other people; an enthusiasm for making plans to improve and an energy to keep going despite a lack of encouragement. It follows that an effective manager is also one who is able to encourage and guide others through this continuous process of self- and professional improvement.

ESTABLISHING YOURSELF AS A MANAGER

Being promoted to a more senior appointment in any occupation is generally a testing experience. Although some of the tasks in the new job will be familiar, there will be new responsibilities and additional tasks. The most difficult transition of all is that from being primarily a practitioner in your profession to become a first line manager.

When a ward sister is promoted from existing staff of a ward she can find a sudden fracture in her existing relationships. Most consider it necessary to become a little distant from former colleagues but without losing touch or undermining an existing friendly relationship. Some go too far in making the separation whilst others try to act as if there had been no change. A complication in trying to make the right relationship can be that of resentment from others.

In one case, a nurse was appointed to the role of team leader in a coronary care unit over two others with higher seniority in the 'off-duty list'. This was justified by her previous experience and personal qualities, but led one of the staff to become aggressive and difficult. The team leader tried to use tact and consideration in the hope of winning her round, but this added extra pressure at a time when she needed the full support of her colleagues.

Another common problem for the newly promoted supervisor is trying to marry the conflicting demands of senior managers and junior staff. Senior nurses usually value a sister who is efficient, well-organised, manages within budget limits, shows initiative, sets high standards and shows a good example. Nurses on the other hand like a sister who is prepared to work alongside them, is available to answer problems, shows clinical expertise, is caring, is supportive, speaks up for staff, keeps them informed and runs interesting teaching sessions.

The tensions that come with additional responsibility will be worst during the first few months in a new post. It can be easier if you have come from another unit in that your authority might be more readily accepted by existing staff. Lack of local knowledge can make it more difficult to identify the minefield of thwarted ambitions, hobby horses and resistance to change that exist in most work places.

It is essential to have resilience and a practical plan to cope with the first few months in a new appointment. There are three key aspects of this:

1. Be prepared for some initial difficulties; do not expect a smooth transition.
2. Expect that these problems will diminish with time as you become more experi-

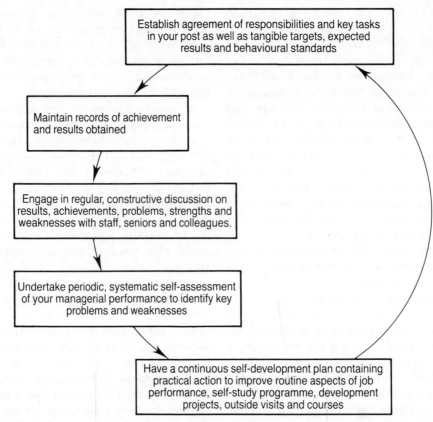

Establish agreement of responsibilities and key tasks
in your post as well as tangible targets, expected
results and behavioural standards

Maintain records of achievement
and results obtained

Engage in regular, constructive discussion on
results, achievements, problems, strengths and
weaknesses with staff, seniors and colleagues.

Undertake periodic, systematic self-assessment
of your managerial performance to identify key
problems and weaknesses

Have a continuous self-development plan containing
practical action to improve routine aspects of job
performance, self-study programme, development
projects, outside visits and courses

Fig. 2.2 Developing management effectiveness. It is possible to start at any point in this cycle and then proceed to the next logical step.

enced and staff adjust to you. Remember a new job is a learning experience.
3. Develop a well-considered 'self-induction' programme so that you can acquire additional knowledge and skills quickly, identify the real problems in a unit and build up constructive relationships with others. The components of such a self-induction plan will include:
   a. Gain knowledge of procedures, systems, rules, policies, working practices and local customs.
   b. Gain an understanding of staff personalities and expectations, whilst seeking to develop co-operative working relationships.
   c. Gain an appreciation of the 'politics' of the organisation.
   d. Maintain the existing working routines of the unit.
   e. Assess the effectiveness of these routines and of the unit staff.
   f. Identify appropriate priorities for improving practices, standards, resources and staff effectiveness from careful assessment and from consultation with those involved.
   g. Identify the appropriate management role in the routine and development actvities of the unit and within the wider context of the hospital/community service.

Before looking in detail at the managerial skills that are needed for personal effectiveness it is useful to consider the context in which managers have to practise their craft — organisations.

REFERENCES

Armstrong M 1981 Practical nurse management. Edward Arnold, London

Clark C C, Shea C A 1979 Management in nursing. McGraw Hill, Maidenhead

Lemin B 1977 First line nursing management. Pitman Medical, Tunbridge Wells

Long A, Harrison S 1985 Health service performance, Croom Helm, London

Marriner A 1984 Guide to nursing. C V Mosby, New York

Matthews A 1982 In charge of the ward, Blackwell Scientific Publications Oxford

Nelson E, Blenkinsop D 1972 Managing the system. Bookstall publications

Pearson A 1983 The clinical nursing unit. William Heinemann, London

Perry E 1978 Ward management and teaching. Baillière Tindall London

Rowden R 1984 Managing nursing. Baillière Tindall, London

Schurr M 1975 Nurses and management. English University Press, Sevenoaks

SECTION TWO

The context of nurse management

3

Organisational structures and theories

Many staff in the NHS are somewhat perplexed by the frequency with which they are afflicted with the upheavals associated with 'reorganisation'. However, such experience of regular changes in the way that authority, job titles and tasks are allocated is not restricted to the Health Service. All large business corporations have regular modifications of their internal structures, as do small growing businesses and public agencies. Large-scale nationalised industries and other major public services have similarly been through the throws of organisational change. This process will continue as those at the top of organisations try to ensure that they adapt to the constant pressures of change in economic, technological and social circumstances.

Although there may be good reasons for regular modification, there is also a need for some reasonably permanent arrangement when people work together so that each undertakes appropriate tasks and that these are co-ordinated into a whole.

The underlying concept behind such arrangements is usually that individuals should have a specific set of tasks which make up an identifiable job and that authority to give instructions and commit resources is delegated in diminishing quantity from the chief executive down to the most junior supervisor. The advantage of a logical framework is that it should be stable and self-perpetuating. Individual members may change but the system continues. There are different forms or shapes that organisational structures can take. There is not one universally right format. Corporate aims, technology, 'market' factors and social considerations will be taken into account by those advising on the most appropriate form.

There is one particularly common structure in large organisations, both in business and the public services. This has been termed a 'bureaucracy' and is the prevailing characteristic of the National Health Service as well as independent health care organisations. Unfortunately the term has come into general use as a condemnation of slow decision-taking and unreasonable adherence to rules and procedures. The word as applied in this context does not imply criticism, however, but is meant to distinguish organisations with some standard characteristics. These can be summarised as:

1. Each employee has a narrow, specialised range of responsibility which can be precisely defined in a written job description.
2. Each employee has one direct superior so that there is a clear line of command from the most senior to the most junior post.
3. Each manager supervises a specific and limited number of subordinates, thus giving close control termed the 'span of control'.
4. Jobs are grouped together into specialised sections and departments under particular managers.
5. Decision-making is centralised within a fixed hierarchy of authority, the pyramid of authority.
6. There are formal rules and procedures for all routine and predictable situations.

If all these features are present in one organisation, this would be an extreme form of bureaucracy. All large organisations will have certain elements of bureaucracy, but there are likely to be some variations according to particular circumstances.

One difference will be the extent of centralisation in management decision-making and

management systems. If the formal rules, standards and procedures are all designed by one individual or small clique, and are binding on all managers and staff with detailed reporting back to this body, the result will be extreme centralised control. This may be an appropriate organisational concept where the 'business' has considerable uniformity and standardisation of product or service. There are some inherent advantages to such centralisation — strict control of resources, great uniformity and avoidance of unnecessary variation or duplication. However, such a system can also be a handicap to the achievement of the goals of an enterprise or public activity. Limited scope for individual initiatives, little willingness to accept responsibility at lower levels, inability to provide diversity of product or service, heavy work load on top managers, lack of flexibility and heavy overhead costs of administration and information systems are the main drawbacks of centralised control.

As a result, some large organisations have made deliberate attempts to decentralise management control. This can be achieved on a geographical basis by creating regions or areas, for which specific objectives are agreed but where local management has autonomy to meet these in ways it thinks best. An alternative form of decentralisation in a business is to set up distinct product divisions or semi-autonomous businesses within a group. Again there will be agreed objectives but greater freedom for management to devise means for meeting these.

Some large companies with apparently decentralised structures will retain some form of centralised control through the functional management activities. In this arrangement each main specialism will have a central director, with staff answering in the regions or divisions. This will ensure that corporate policies and procedures are maintained in such areas as personnel, research, public relations etc. Such arrangements can be consistent with local autonomy, however, as these functions are only advisory at the centre and functional staff are directly responsible to general management in each division or region.

A completely decentralised organisation, then, is one where the sub-units are able to develop as separate, multi-functional 'costs and profit' centres under their own general management, working towards targets that have been negotiated with central management or the directors of the parent company.

Thus, large organisations can be composed of one centrally controlled bureaucracy, or a number of semi-independent units which may also be run on bureaucratic principles, only on a smaller scale. The significant features of this form of organising work are a permanent framework of relationships, jobs, rules and procedures that are intended to co-ordinate efforts of individuals to function like a well-oiled machine. Hence, another term that is applied to describe this system is 'mechanistic'. Although there are many well-recognised advantages in this approach to work organisation, there are some equally well-acknowledged problems. These are summarised in the following table:

Advantages	Disadvantages
1. Individuals have clear guidelines for their work	There is little room for individual initiative
2. Individuals have clearly defined responsibility and authority	Individuals may have only a limited commitment to their work
3. Each individual has one immediate superior	Top management may be too authoritarian
4. Individuals are protected from unfair treatment by the rules and procedures	Too much buck passing and apathy in the middle ranks
5. Individuals have reasonable job security	Rules become inflexible and restrictive
6. High level of efficiency is possible when work is of a predictable nature	Not readily responsive to change

The most significant advantage of a bureaucratic system of organisation is overall efficiency in dealing with large volumes of work. The greatest drawback is difficulty in adapting to changing circumstances and local variation.

Where there is sufficient pressure for greater flexibility there may be a response from within the organisations. Individuals or groups of staff act to bend the rules informally and to bypass official rules or procedures as this becomes the only way to achieve results. It is common therefore to find two organisational structures. One is official or 'formal', as shown on any published organisation chart; the other is the 'informal' arrangement of how an organisation actually works in practice. Such informal structures are present in all large bureaucracies as the practical response from responsible members trying to meet the changing circumstances in which they have to function.

It is possible for top management to adopt means that are intended to find ways of modifying the formal systems. They can provide the impetus for interdepartmental working parties, special 'task teams' and 'project groups' to investigate problems that cannot be resolved through the normal channels and to make recommendations for change. Such schemes involve the temporary grouping of staff drawn from several specialisms that cut across the normal command structures. Such arrangements can be termed 'adhocracy'.

Within such task teams there should be no status differences, authority will come from individual expertise rather than formal position. The method of working will be flexible and co-operative as required by the particular problems being investigated. With this approach an organisation can function on bureaucratic lines for routine activities whilst having a range of adhoc working parties engaged on a variety of developmental tasks in an attempt to promote innovation from within.

It is possible to take 'adhocracy' further. In large organisations some specialist sections will have to work on a permanent adhoc basis. If their normal work is concerned with 'one off' projects it is more efficient to arrange for people to work in changeable groups and to fulfil different levels of responsibility in each.

It would be usual for such departments as management services, data processing, building services, training, research and development to be set up in this manner. The ultimate extreme of an adhocracy is found in such industries as construction consultancy and aviation development. It is necessary in such businesses to have several major projects on the go at the same time. These will often be in different stages of completion and of differing scales. This means that staff may have to be allocated to more than one project at a time, or having finished a contribution to one will have to move into another part of the business to start work on a new project. Such organisations may have a permanent framework in a hierarchical, pyramid form but imposed on this will be temporary arrangements to second individuals on to priority work not directly supervised by their permanent superior. The formal device that enables individuals to be allocated to different working groups or various work tasks at the same time but also ensuring some efficient co-ordination of the whole is a 'Matrix' system (see Fig. 3.1). Organisations which have been deliberately set up to respond to varying demand can be called 'organic' as opposed to the more rigid 'mechanistic' organisations.

The answer to the fundamental question, 'What is the best form of organisational structure?' is one usually given in response to other queries about the best approach to management: 'It all depends on . . . .'. There is no ideal model for running a business or public service. The circumstances which will have a bearing on deciding whether a centralised bureaucracy or a decentralised matrix organisation is most appropriate are the demands of 'customers', the nature of the 'market', the technology employed, the type of staff employed, and the financial constraints.

A possible solution to the problem of centralisation or decentralisation for the manufacturing industry is a hybrid structure. This arrangement will have semi-autonomous product groups or business activities run by a general manager and a team of line and functional specialists reporting financial returns to a central management board. There will also be an advisory reporting link between the various specialist managers across the whole organisation. Thus there may be a production managers' committee, a personnel managers' committee etc. chaired by the appropriate head office director. These committees are intended to share expertise and generally raise standards of management in the various professional groups. The functional directors may also be responsible for the professional and career development of senior staff in one clear function across the whole company.

Thus the hybrid organisation depends on dual reporting, or even multiple reporting where managers are also involved in inter-departmental project groups or task teams. This may present some conflict of interest and ambiguity but these can be managed constructively with proper support and training for middle and junior managers.

Although there is little that middle or junior managers can do to alter the fundamental character of the organisation in which they are employed, it is essential to have an informed understanding of its basic structure and the trends in various re-organisations. This understanding will suggest the limits to personal autonomy and the difficulties or otherwise of being personally innovative.

Such an overview of your place of employment is as relevant for a ward sister/charge nurse as it is for a director of nursing services or a senior manager in a commercial enterprise.

ORGANISATIONAL CULTURE

There is a danger in presenting general prescriptions on how effective managers should act. This can lead to the wrong assumption that successful managers can be transferred from job to job, from organisation to organisation and always remain successful as the skills of managing are the same, whatever the nature of a business.

The error here is in ignoring the clearly observable differences in the nature of various

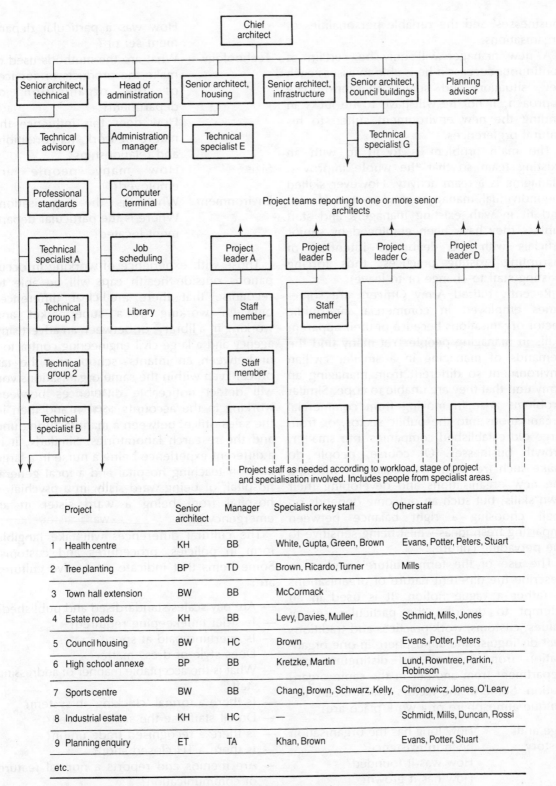

	Project	Senior architect	Manager	Specialist or key staff	Other staff
1	Health centre	KH	BB	White, Gupta, Green, Brown	Evans, Potter, Peters, Stuart
2	Tree planting	BP	TD	Brown, Ricardo, Turner	Mills
3	Town hall extension	BW	BB	McCormack	
4	Estate roads	KH	BB	Levy, Davies, Muller	Schmidt, Mills, Jones
5	Council housing	BW	HC	Brown	Evans, Potter, Peters
6	High school annexe	BP	BB	Kretzke, Martin	Lund, Rowntree, Parkin, Robinson
7	Sports centre	BW	BB	Chang, Brown, Schwarz, Kelly,	Chronowicz, Jones, O'Leary
8	Industrial estate	KH	HC	—	Schmidt, Mills, Duncan, Rossi
9	Planning enquiry	ET	TA	Khan, Brown	Evans, Potter, Stuart
	etc.				

Fig. 3.1 Use of matrix management within a local authority department.

'businesses' and the variable personalities of organisations.

A new manager will only be certain of continuous success if he is able to assess each new situation and select an appropriate approach; if not he will have to be lucky in finding the new environment suited to his natural preferences.

The main problem is to fit in with an existing team so that the whole improves. Managing is a team activity. However skilled the individual, managers need to complement and fit in with existing managers and staff (unless they have been employed by senior officials with the deliberate intention of disrupting existing practices, thus forcing existing staff to change or to leave).

Recently retired Army Officers are sometimes employed in commercial or public sector organisations because of their apparent skills in managing people. Yet many find the demands of managing in a smaller civilian environment so different from managing an army unit that they are unable to cope. Similar problems arise in moving from commercial organisations into the public sector, or from large old established companies into smaller, growth businesses. Of course, people do make such transitions successfully, enriching the new organisations and developing their own skills, but such an outcome depends on their choosing a right balance between imparting fresh ideas whilst being sensitive to the pervading culture.

The use of the term 'culture' applied to describe the different nature of organisations is rather a vague notion. It is used in an attempt to describe the particular set of values, customs, work practices and traditions that distinguish the atmosphere in one organisation from another and distinguish one department from another in the same organisation. Some of the factors which create the unique atmosphere of a work place are:

Age and history	How long has the organisation been in existence?
	How was it founded?
	How has it grown?
	How was a particular department set up?
Technology	What are the methods used to make the products or services of the organisation or department?
	How does this influence the nature of work, its conditions and relationships?
Size	How many people are employed?
Environment	Where is the organisation? Where is the particular department located?

Those with experience of working in occupations outside health care will be able to recognise that there are clear differences between working in a supermarket and working in a library, or between an advertising agency and a large civil engineering contractor, or between an infants' school and the tax office. Even within the same organisations you will detect noticeable differences between working in the accounts section and then in the sales office, between a manufacturing unit and the research laboratories. Similarly, it is a different experience being a nurse in a large London teaching hospital and a local general hospital, or being ward sister in a psychiatric hospital from being a ward sister in an emergency unit.

The cultural differences will take tangible form in policies, procedures and customs. Some items that indicate alternative cultures are:

— Are pay scales standardised and published?
— Is strict timekeeping required?
— Is overtime paid at specific rates?
— Does style of dress matter?
— What is the acceptable manner of addressing staff?
— Is there a formal 'clocking' in system?
— Do all staff use the same canteen?
— Is there a recognised trade union?
— Is there a TU closed shop?
— Are memos and reports a normal feature of communication?

— Have all staff been through a standard training programme?
— Is there a published organisational chart?
— Are there official job descriptions?

In many 'high technology' businesses dress is casual, the average age is young, qualifications amongst professional staff are high. Use of first names is common and staff will be expected to consult directly with each other to resolve technical problems. In older, larger, more bureaucratic organisations it is common to find greater variety of professional background, more formality in style and greater protocol in contact between different sections of the organisation.

These observations may seem so obvious as to be hardly worth mentioning. Obvious they may be, but the significance for managers can be considerable.

A manager recruited from a small and loosely structured organisation into one with greater formality may find it hard to be effective if he has been used to quick access to decision-makers and informal reference to a network of professional contacts. A personnel manager recruited by a small but rapidly expanding electronics company from a large manufacturer may be tempted to introduce more precise systems for recruitment, salary administration, appraisal, discipline etc. which may be rejected by the more technology-oriented professional staff.

Clearly, there are implications for managers in health care. The pressures to change organisational structures in the NHS have come from outside influences, and in many ways have been intended to change organisational culture towards being more cost and efficiency conscious.

It is to be expected that considerable internal resistence should arise from existing professionals. The strategy of the Griffith Report (1983) included recommendations not only that new posts of general managers should be created but that many of these could be filled by people with managerial experience outside the NHS. The resulting tensions are evident from the resignation of the Chairman of the NHS management board in 1986 and other well-publicised disputes between staff and new general managers.

The promotion of health care professionals to more senior appointments should not involve such great problems of transition. The particular difficulties of nurses taking up their first managerial post are discussed in Chapter 2. At this point it should be clear that, even with first-hand knowledge of the Health Service, senior nurses should take account of the particular organisational culture when they move from one hospital to another or if they move from the NHS into the independent sector.

REFERENCES

Griffith Report 1983 NHS management enquiry. HMSO, London
Handy C 1976 Understanding organisations. Penguin Books, London
Stewart R 1967 The reality of management. Pan Books, London

4

Management of health care organisations

THE STRUCTURE

It should be apparent from the general descriptions in the previous chapter that both the National Health Service and the independent hospital groups are essentially bureaucratic organisations, although there may be variations in the degree of centralisation and many deliberate attempts to foster the review and development of improvements through the medium of 'ad hoc' working parties and project teams. The main reason for this form of organisation is the need to ensure that appropriate standards and procedures for treating patients are delivered in all parts of a health care service.

The essential bureaucratic framework of the NHS was established when the Service first came under state control. The overall aim of the NHS has remained that of providing an equal service to the whole population, considering the quality of care available and the access to that care. Although there have been several reorganisations in the NHS and some criticism of the centralised control, the fundamentally bureaucratic structure has remained as described in the 1972 DHSS publication, *Management Arrangements for the Reorganised NHS*:

1. Responsibility should be clearly defined and allocated.
2. There should be a clear executive hierarchy in which delegation downwards is matched by accountability upwards.

Since its inception there has also been a continuous pressure towards centralisation of management control. The various architects of the structure have tried to resolve the fundamental dilemma of having sufficient centralisation to ensure the equal provision and access to health care for the whole community, whilst leaving some local autonomy to respond to the needs of a particular local community.

The fact that most funds of the NHS are provided by central government and that there has to be some overall planning for the delivery of an egalitarian service will lead towards centralised accountability. Ideally such a service needs to recognise the differences in local need and demand and allow participation by the public at the local level. However, as medicine is a limited resource of a highly specialised and increasingly technological nature, it is not easy for the public to know what it should choose for the various options available. Thus most of the decisions about provision are taken by medical experts, based on their views of the best fit between public needs and the resources available.

The NHS has been described as a 'professional bureaucracy' in which the medical experts have a high degree of control over the use of resources and delivery of services, despite the ultimate responsibility of the Secretary of State to Parliament for every penny that is spent.

The present framework of the Health Service (1986) is really based on rearrangements in 1974 of the original structure, and was intended to achieve an appropriate balance between those conflicting dilemmas. This was explained in proposals first published by DHSS in 1972.

The area health authorities will be responsible for achieving national health care objectives through the provision of comprehensive health services designed to meet the demands of communities within districts.

The result was a three-tiered structure of administration made up of 15 regional health authorities responsible directly to the Secretary of State for Health and Social Services; 90 area health authorities responsible to the appropriate regions; and then 200 separate health districts under these area authorities. The intention was for the district to be the basic local health care organisation serving the needs of a population between 200 000 and 500 000. This local organisation was co-ordinated by a multi-disciplinary team — the district management team (DMT) which had representatives of the main local interest groups and was required to work out a concensus for decision-making. The membership of the DMT was defined as:

— Three doctors (hospital consultant, general practitioner and community physician)
— The chief nurse (district nursing officer)
— The chief administrator (district administrator)
— The accountant (district treasurer)

Under this arrangement the NHS did not have any general manager or chief executive posts under whom the hierarchy of line and functional management was to converge. The overall structure made up of DMTs, area authorities, area teams of officers, regional authorities, regional teams of officers, extensive functional management, community health councils, family practitioner committees, chairman of the various levels of authority and administrators, was criticised on several counts. One was complexity.

In 1979 a Royal Commission reviewed the working of the 1974 structure and confirmed the main critical points, particularly the number of tiers, the large number of administrators, the slow decision-making, wasted money, poor staff morale and too much functional management. The result was a government consultative paper in 1979 with four main proposals for change (Merrison Report, 1979)

1. To strengthen management arrangements at local level with greater delegation of responsibility to those in the hospital and community services
2. To simplify the structure in England by removing the area tier, and the establishment of district health authorities

3. To simplify the professional advisory services
4. To simplify the planning system.

There were several comments regarding the need to improve the quality of local management, but the possibility of appointing chief executives as the means to achieve this end was rejected. The DMT was to remain the basic management unit supported by the community health councils and a variety of health care planning teams, some of which would be permanently established (elderly, mentally ill etc.) whilst others would be formed on an ad hoc basis.

This modified structure was introduced into practice during 1982. In February 1983, however, the Secretary of State asked a small team of outside business experts to reconsider the NHS structure. As a result, some modifications to the new model were recommended in the Griffith Report (1983). The main thrust seemed to be aimed at changing the existing 'professional bureaucracy' into a more business style professional management organisation. Several new bodies were introduced with the intention of facilitating greater efficiency. A Health Services Supervisory Board was appointed to review the purpose, objectives and direction of the whole NHS; to approve budgets and resources allocation; to make strategic decisions and receive reports on performance and evaluation. The membership of the Board consists of:

— The Secretary of State for Health and Social Security (Chairman)
— The Minister of State for Health
— The Permanent Secretary at the DHSS
— The Chief Medical Officer
— The Chairman of the Management Board
— Two or three additional members with general management skills
— The Chief Nurse.

The inclusion of the Chief Nurse was not in the original Griffith Report but came about as the result of representations from the nursing profession. This new management arrange-

ment was introduced during 1985 and was accompanied by several other changes recommended by Griffith. The Supervisory Board is a part-time monitoring body to which a main executive board reports. The aim of the lower Management Board is to plan the implementation of policies approved by the Supervisory Board, to control performance in the NHS and to give leadership to NHS management. The Board membership consists of:

— The Chairman and Chief Executive
— The Director of Health Authorities
— The Director of Planning and Information Technology
— The Director of Health Authority Liaison
— The Director of Operations
— The Director of Finance
— The Director of Personnel.

There are 14 regional health authorities reporting directly to the Management Board. Each region has the freedom to devise the actual executive body that will have full-time responsibility for overseeing the provision of services for the various district authorities in their locality. These regional bodies are called the regional executive and replace the previous regional team of officers. The proposed structure of each executive has to be approved by the Minister of Health. Thus there is provision for different regions to make variations on the pattern of posts found on the Management Board. The North West Thames Regional Health Authority created a new executive in 1985 with a membership of eight:

— Regional General Manager
— Director of Clinical and Scientific Services
— Director of Finance and Computing
— Director of Planning and Information
— Director of Personnel
— Director of Support Services
— Regional Nursing Director
— Director of Estate Development.

In the case of the North West Thames RHA the Regional General Manager was previously Regional Administrator and the majority of the directors were previously regional officers. In some regions the general manager and other directors were appointed from outside the NHS.

One of the most significant changes in the philosophy of management in the Griffith proposals was a move from concensus team management to that of having the ultimate responsibility for the delivery of an effective health care service resting with the new post of general manager. At a national level, the Chief Executive of the Management Board is the most senior appointment in the NHS. Similarly, at regional level the general manager is the role of chief executive.

In this 1985 reorganisation the health districts become district health authorities with a district general manager as chief executive. Again some autonomy existed for each authority to devise a structure that best suited its local circumstances, although there has been a tendency for the structure at regional level to be reflected at district level.

Incorporated into this district structure are a number of units with a management team responsible for achieving objectives agreed for a particular part of health care provision locally. A common arrangement is for three such units to be set up in a district — acute unit, community unit and the psychiatric unit — with a general manager co-ordinating the efforts of the unit team and reporting to the district general manager. There are also a number of health care planning teams to advise the DMT directly as well as the continuation of community health councils.

The most significant change as far as nurse managers at ward level are concerned, is the creation of unit management consisting of a senior nurse, a doctor and an administrator reporting to a single unit general manager. The advantage of this arrangement should be twofold. One is the access to speedier decision-making at local level and clearer accountability. The other is the possible career opening provided by unit general manager appointments to which many nurses will be able to aspire.

MANAGEMENT ISSUES IN THE NHS

The various attempts to modify the overall structure of the NHS have been carried out to find the best compromise between providing a national service to meet the health problems of the whole population and the need for stringent cost control to ensure value for money, whilst incorporating the advances in medical technology and treatment. There are several major issues that have to be recognised in considering how effective the management arrangements for the NHS are likely to be.

The sheer size of the enterprise is a major problem in seeking some central control without undermining local autonomy too severely. A brief statement of some general statistics gives an indication of the massive scale of the NHS:

— The NHS owns 2600 hospitals with 450 000 beds.
— 6 million inpatients are treated annually.
— 37 million outpatients are treated annually.
— The NHS employs 38 000 doctors and 415 000 nurses covering 36 specialities.
— The NHS employs 211 000 ancillary workers and 113 000 administrators and clerical staff.
— In total the NHS employs some 1 million staff.

A second unique managerial problem in the NHS is the employment of a wide range of medical professions, all with a varying degree of independence in their training and professional code of conduct, but all of whom have to be co-ordinated to function effectively within the cost restraints imposed by Parliament to provide the best standard of health care possible.

The third unusual feature in the NHS is the role of the customers and 'clients.' In most businesses, including the nationalised industries, the customer has a significant impact on the type of service provided and therefore indirectly on the managerial structure. The reason for the powerful influence of customers is that they are the main source of income and therefore have to be satisfied if they are not to take their custom elsewhere. Generally in the NHS, patients and the general public have less powerful influences in not being a source of income and for most having no real alternative source of supply. Thus it can be argued that the structure has been developed to meet the needs of centralised bureaucratic control and problems of meeting the needs of various professional interest groups.

The reorganisations emerging from the Griffith Report were another attempt to find the most workable solution to the inherent conflicts and dilemmas of the NHS.

There has been a problem in the past in determining who actually manages the Health Service: the health care professionals or the civil servants and NHS administrators? Now in theory at least, the general managers at unit, district, region and national level have the ultimate management responsibility and authority. In practice, it may be difficult for general managers to exercise real power in the face of the dominating influence of health care professionals.

For senior nurses and ward sisters there has always been a significant problem in working out their hierarchical relationship with doctors and understanding who really are the line managers in a hospital or community service. For nurse managers in the 1980s this problem will remain, and it is important for them to appreciate the underlying organisational issues involved.

Nurses are the largest occupational group in the Health Service and, together with doctors, have the greatest direct responsibility for the delivery of patient care. Traditionally these two occupational groups have been arranged in a separate hierarchy with their own line management structures.

Doctors or managers?

This arrangement of doctors in a hospital has been described as 'a firm' and is made up of as many as five grades, diminishing in

seniority from the consultant, senior registrar, registrar, senior house officer to house officer. In theory, this structure requires a consultant to be responsible ultimately for his or her patients, making final decisions about their treatment and then delegating various responsibilities to the other doctors in the team according to their abilities.

There has been a long running debate about the way doctors function in the health service, the dilemma being whether they are part of the management or whether they are independent, professional workers giving most of their time to practising within the NHS arrangements. Clearly, a consultant has considerable authority to direct the work of doctors in his 'Firm' and to monitor their effectiveness, and therefore could be regarded as the line manager for this group. Further than this, doctors, and especially consultants, have a major say in the way services are developed locally and how resources are allocated. One difficulty in simply regarding consultants as senior managers and other doctors as middle and junior managers is their professional accountability.

Throughout the history of the NHS, doctors have acted to preserve their professional autonomy. This means that they are ultimately responsible for their clinical decisions and actions to the General Medical Council. Thus whilst having an overwhelming influence on what actually happens in the hospital service they have not had to accept the managerial consequences of this influence.

There have been several attempts to better integrate doctors into the management structure. In the 1974 reorganisation, doctors were involved in the basic unit of health service management, the district management team. There was considerable criticism, however, of their role, in particular that they were often not really integrated members but tended to use their veto to protect their own interests. In the Griffith Report of 1983 there was significant comment about this ambiguous position of doctors and recommendations that they should become a real part of the formal management structure.

Doctors must accept the managerial responsibility that goes with clinical freedom
(Griffith Report 1983)

The way of achieving this aim in practice remains difficult at regional or district level, and is unlikely to remove the persistent problem of ambiguity in the relationships between doctors, nurse managers and nurses at the ward level. This problem leads many nurses to resent the manner and assumptions of some of the medical staff they have to deal with. Ideally, the relationship should be one of professional partnership working in the interests of better patient care. The conflict is well summarised in one study (Buehler 1977) which found two significant differences in perception between nurses' and doctors' views:

. . . . it was found that the doctor saw the nurse as working 'under' him, and the nurse saw herself as working 'with' the physician.

. . . . The nurses feel they are training to exercise judgement whereas the doctors expect nurses to be obedient extensions of their own professional judgement.

Nurses as managers

In considering the place of nurse managers in the overall structure of the Health Service there is much less ambiguity. All nurses are employed by a particular health authority, although subject to a code of professional ethics formulated in the UKCC.

They can be dismissed as normal employees of the health authority. Clearly, most nurse posts are directly concerned with applying medical treatments and giving advice to patients and the general public. The senior nurse posts, with a responsibility for planning, organising and monitoring the work of such nursing staff, are therefore part of the line management in a health service. It is possible within the various grades of senior nurse appointments to distinguish between those that are supervisory, those that are middle and those that are senior management in emphasis.

First line or supervisory managers in the hospital sector are the ward sister/charge nurse posts. The primary aim is to ensure that proper medical care is delivered to a specific group of patients and any problems that arise from achieving this day by day, shift by shift, are resolved. There should be a change in priority in posts higher up the grades of senior nurse involving direct control over a number of ward sisters. Whilst there is concern that the daily arrangement for providing adequate nursing care is functioning properly, there should be greater emphasis on developing staff, planning and allocating resources, communicating and liaising with other sections in the hospital — all tasks associated with middle management roles in large organisations.

Senior posts in the hierarchy of line nurse management include those of assistant director of nursing services and director of nursing services. Here the emphasis should change towards more long-term planning, overall allocation of resources, monitoring the schemes of development for staff and resources, making sure that senior nurses play a proper management role in leading their teams of ward sisters and trying to achieve proper co-ordination with all other sectors of the hospital.

Administrators and specialists

One of the attempts to make an effective organisation in which doctors, nurses and other professional health care staff can be properly co-ordinated, was the introduction of administrators in direct line from the DHSS down to the district levels. The administrator could be held responsible for the implementation of plans and controls to achieve the objectives of a National Health Service. This arrangement was extensively questioned by those inside the service and the various authorities who have been charged with reviewing the structural arrangements.

The paradox of the NHS is that while it is the professional experts (doctors, nurses and other service providers) who decide which patient gets what in the way of treatment, the machinery of accountability is designed only to make the bureaucratic experts (administrators and civil servants) answerable for what he or she does.

(Barnard & Lee 1977)

Another issue of management in the structure of the NHS between 1974 and 1984 was the relatively fast growth of functional management and 'professionalism'. There was a tendency for such posts as personnel, suppliers, catering, buildings, management and services officers to be found at district, area and regional level as well as physiotherapy, occupational therapy and other professional structure, and for each department to acquire a certain independence from the rest of the service.

The 1982 reorganisation and the 1983 Griffith proposals were implemented in response to these major issues and problems in the NHS management arrangements. Thus, removal of the area level organisation, the reduction of functionalism and the introduction of the general manager concept were expected to improve the standards of management. It will be some years before it is clear whether these changes have achieved this objective.

It is clear however that senior nurses and ward level nurse managers will need to develop greater management skills in order to maintain their influence in management decision-making and to maintain a creditable relationship with general managers and medical staff. Having briefly examined the general theories relating to management and organisation, and considered the ways in which such theories have been applied in the various models for organising the NHS, it is appropriate to turn to the main topics of this book, 'What management skills are relevant to nurse managers?'

REFERENCES

Barnard K, Lee K 1977 Conflicts in the National Health Service. Croom Helm, London

Buehler J 1977 Nurses and physicians in transition. MI Research Press: Bowker Publishing, Epping

Consumers' Association 1983 A patient's guide to the NHS. Hodder and Stoughton, Sevenoaks

Department of Health and Social Security 1972 Management arrangements for the reorganised NHS. HMSO, London

Dimmock S 1985 Griffith and NHS nurse management. Nursing Times, January 23rd and February 6th.

Gatherer A, Warren M 1971 Management and the health services. Pergamon Press, Oxford

Illiffe S 1983 The NHS: A picture of health, Lawrence and Wishart, London

Jaques E 1978 Health services. Heinemann, London

Klien R 1983 The politics of the National Health Service. Longman, Harlow

NHS Management enquiry 1983 Griffith Report. HMSO, London

Merrison Report 1979 Royal Commission on the NHS. HMSO, London

SECTION **THREE**

Management
skills for
nurse managers

5

Planning techniques

Successful planning is the basis of all effective management. It is the link between what you want to achieve and actual achievement. Planning is the process of assessing what activities and resources are required and then organising the means of bringing together these resources and activities in the most efficient way. Thus planning is essential at all levels of health care.

It is needed by the National Health Service Management Board to ensure that overall organisational aims are fulfilled, and is similarly required by regional and district health authority senior management. It is necessary at hospital, unit and ward level to ensure resources are available and that work is carried out efficiently, as well as being required at a personal level by managers and staff to ensure their own efforts are effective. Finally, but most importantly, planning is essential for the effective treatment of individual patients.

The more senior the level of management the longer is the time-scale of planning. The true function of national and regional staff within the NHS, or directors in the independent sector, is to undertake 'corporate or strategic planning'. This should be concerned with assessing demand and capacity for health care in the community, devising strategies and developing resources needed to meet these needs in the long term (more than two years) and possibly the medium term (three months to two years). This requires effective fore-

43

casting to take account of likely changes in the nature of the population, probable demand for health services and likely changes in medical and clinical practice. This will lead to broad decisions about the need to increase or decrease the number of hospital beds, decisions to build premises and decisions to extend or decrease resources for community care. Thus a corporate plan might indicate an intention of building a new hospital, closing wards in existing hospitals, extending screening facilities and increasing provision for community-based treatment.

Such long-term and medium-term planning in the public services is clearly linked to particular government policy on public expenditure and economic planning in general. As such decisions have considerable impact on future employment prospects, trade unions and professional institutes have a wish to influence the direction of planning decisions. Even without formal trade union involvement the final formation of corporate plans will not take place without considerable input from management and professional staff and various outside interest groups. Thus the final result will be a merging of 'planning from the top down' and 'planning from the bottom up', with some account of consumer and community interests.

In each tier of health authority management there will be concern with implementing overall strategic plans and concern in making medium- and short-term (less than three months) plans.

This description of the processes of organisational planning for a public service is very idealised. In practice there are ambiguities, conflicts, professional jealousies, political pressures, errors in forecasting and overall uncertainty that make long-term planning especially difficult. Another issue which causes concern in planning is not so much the accuracy of plans but the appropriate role for senior management. There is often criticism of senior managers in centralised organisations that they tend to be over-involved with short-term plans and operational problems instead of delegating these to middle manage-

ment. When this happens, senior managers either become over-burdened with work or are so concerned with short-term issues that they neglect the more distant planning requirements. Strategic planning in public sector organisations can be especially hazardous as senior managers and senior government officials find that politicians make arbitrary changes in previously agreed plans, or get too involved in the means of achieving corporate aims.

Despite these problems, nurse managers at all levels need to understand what strategic and operational plans (or lack of plans) influence their particular part of health care, as well as being able to make a competent contribution to planning activities of this aspect of the service. Most important of all is the need to apply the techniques of simple planning to their own areas of responsibility and their own activities. It is this aspect that we consider in more detail in the rest of this chapter.

UNIT PLANNING

A senior nurse as a planner has to make the best arrangements she can to organise resources required to provide patient care in an effective manner. In theory, the level of demand for nursing services and the requirement for satisfactory treatment should be assessed first to determine the resource allocation and answer the basis question, 'what do we need to provide a satisfactory service?'

There are many practical difficulties in such 'capacity planning' to service health care activities; one is the dilemma involved in trying to fit often unpredictable demand into a fixed routine and a strictly limited level of staffing. This is most evident in emergency units or health centre surgeries. There have been a number of studies on such problems using some of the quantitative techniques of operational research. The aim is to find the optimum practical level of resource to meet a particular situation. Thus, an overnight ward might have a range of demand from a minimum of one to a maximum of ten patients. To equip and staff for the maximum would be excessively costly, to only have near the minimum would be failing to provide the necessary services.

Another problem in resourcing health care is that large numbers of patients have to receive treatments of varying duration from specialist staff or equipment, but have to wait until this is available. Thus there is the 'queueing' problem. Again, a considerable number of studies have been made using various quantitative techniques.

Basically, the decision in commercial activities is that of whether the cost of providing more resources and a speedier service will be offset by greater income from customers who are prevented from using alternative suppliers. In the public hospital the problem is not that of 'customers' finding alternative suppliers, but that of excessive patient queues for admission being contrary to the aims of the NHS. Many patients, once admitted, spend time in beds 'queueing' to be treated, to be seen by a consultant or to be discharged. If such queues could be reduced by smoothing out bottle-necks, or increasing resources in selected areas, this would release beds and so reduce waiting lists. Thus the application of mathematical or computer modelling techniques to such issues is as relevant in health care as it is in a large retail store or a batch production engineering company.

In the independent hospital sector, commercial considerations will be more relevant; reducing unnecessary queues will either enable the price of treatment to patients to be reduced or prevent unnecessary loss of income from potential patients going elsewhere.

There are further difficulties in estimating the level of staff required to provide nursing care. In practice, there is often disagreement between senior nurses and general managers or unit administrators on what constitutes the 'work' or nursing care. There are obvious manual and clinical activities about which there is little debate, but it is argued that the nurse's role involves advising, informing and

comforting patients as an essential part of care. These activities are harder to quantify and are subject to debate.

As a result of these difficulties, many nurse managers will have to approach capacity planning in another way, accepting the level of resources available and deciding the best way to allocate these. 'What is the best we can do with what we've got?'. Every planning activity, however, requires a manager to adopt a logical approach and a willingness to search for better methods of organising work tasks.

Most newly promoted senior nurses will inherit a working unit. In a hospital ward the routine events (such as doctors' rounds, admissions, discharges, operation days/times, visitors, waking, meals, bedmaking, medicine, temperature, pulse, respiration, therapy, toilet, bathing, cleaning, lights out, etc.) will have an established routine and staffing pattern. From time to time there is a need to undertake a critical review of existing arrangements, or to plan afresh for a new unit or service. In these circumstances it can be helpful to follow a four stage technique used for 'process planning'.

Stage one

The 'planner manager', or planning team, should clarify the nature of the patient service (surgical ward, family planning clinic, emergency unit, etc.) or administration service (staff recruitment, inservice training, etc.) to be provided, or items to be made if it concerns a 'production' unit.

Stage two

Planners try to outline the alternative methods of delivering the treatments, providing service or making items. This can be approached in two steps. First identify the basic activities required.

Activity 1. Admit patient to ward
2. Patient records obtained
3. Interview patient
4. Prepare individual nursing plan

5. Plan approved
6. Plan retained in the office etc.

Next look at each activity to consider how this might be carried out in practice, noting several possible alternatives.

Activity 1. Admission procedure by ward receptionist or, senior nurse on duty, or junior nurse
2. Patient record accompany patient, or receptionist obtains record from medical records department
3. Record passed to nurse; or examined by sister
4. Patient interviewed immediately; or at specific time by staff nurse; or junior nurse
5. Individual plan prepared by staff nurse; or by junior; then referred to sister.

Stage three

Planners evaluate the alternative methods and the logic of the activity sequence. Initially take out the more obvious 'non runners', then do a more detailed analysis of practical aspects, costs involved, value to patient, preference of staff for each alternative.

Stage four

Planners make the final decision on the best process to follow in organising a system to achieve the aims identified in Stage one. The result should be recorded as 'Standard process'.

Clearly this method has been used in designing treatments and procedures which are contained in such manuals as 'Major Accident Procedure Book' or documented as 'Procedure for Voluntary Patient Discharge', but is equally applicable to planning routines in wards, clinics, surgeries etc.

A logical process plan will indicate the detailed activities and tasks required and thus form the basis of either estimating the capacity (staff, materials and equipment) needed to complete these activities in the

required sequence, or to allocate existing capacity. The simplest approach to this is to make lists.

One list should indicate the main items of work to be completed in a month/week/shift (according to the type of work to be planned). This is 'loading' in planning jargon. A second shows the staff available to undertake the work, and a third gives the materials and equipment needed to treat patients, advise clients, etc. The first two lists can be joined by using a simple matrix; the planning task then is to allocate tasks to individuals in the form of ticks on a 'bar chart'. This is called 'scheduling'. The third list will form inventories of stock to be ordered and equipment to purchase, hire or borrow, in what quantities and at what times.

This process is logical but over-simplified. There are many practical difficulties which need to be considered.

For many the 'scheduling' stage will prove to be most difficult as there are insufficient resources to carry out the tasks in the preferred time, in sequence to an adequate standard. Unfilled staff nurse posts, senior staff lacking flexibility, the need to incorporate learning experiences for trainees and staff sickness, are some of the factors which can deplete a nursing establishment, which might be considered inadequate to start with. Thus the art of scheduling requires the use of

Means to increase available staff	Means to decrease available staff
Work overtime	Stop overtime
Borrow staff	Lend staff
Alter holidays/rest days	Give holidays/rest days
Reduce breaks	Send away for training
Reduce absenteeism	More on job training
Work with 'thinner cover'	More breaks
Do priority tasks only	Work slower
Pass work to 'non staff' (volunteers, relatives)	Give higher quality
Patients do more for themselves	Delegate administrative tasks
Staff work harder	Do temporary tasks for other units
Seniors 'act down'	Remove temporary staff
Take on temporary staff	Reduce establishment
Recruit full-time staff	Redeploy

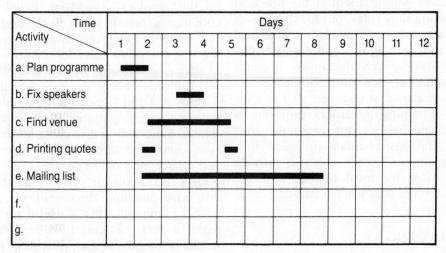

Staff \ Activity	AH	NB	TY	KJ	LP	TM	KI	LL
1	✓		✓					
2		✓						
3	✓		✓					
4				✓	✓	✓		
5		✓					✓	
6								✓
7								✓

Time \ Activity	Days											
	1	2	3	4	5	6	7	8	9	10	11	12
a. Plan programme	▬											
b. Fix speakers			▬									
c. Find venue			▬▬▬▬									
d. Printing quotes		▬			▬							
e. Mailing list		▬▬▬▬▬▬▬▬										
f.												
g.												

Fig. 5.1 A bar chart for planning.

tactics to overcome the mismatch between staff required and staff available.

Some of the common approaches used by ward sisters are included on page 46.

Thus practical scheduling of work will partly be the 'art of the possible' influenced by underlying views of managers on how work should be divided between staff. It has been suggested (Pembrey 1980) that there are four different systems for arranging work in a hospital ward:

1. Allocate nurses to specific tasks (dressings, drugs, etc.) across the whole ward (job assignment or task allocation).
2. Allocate nurses to one section of a ward to undertake varied duties there (part or half ward allocation).
3. Allocate nurses to be fully responsible for selected patients, to plan and carry out an individual care plan (patient assignment).
4. Allocate nurses in pairs/teams of seniors and juniors together to one section of a ward to undertake individual care plans for the very sick, and cover the rest by job assignment (group patient assignment).

The choice will be affected by the demands of the speciality of the ward balanced against what is believed to be best for patients, best for staff and practically possible. There has been considerable advocation of the benefits to patients of more individual attention which is claimed to give nurses increased professional job satisfaction. This has to be offset against an alternative view that fragmenting the tasks of nurses relieves stress and anxiety or the danger of nurses being less flexible, not being prepared to help with needs of patients who 'aren't my patients'. There may also be gains in productivity by staff carrying out repetitive tasks across the whole ward.

Given agreement within a nurse management team on the fundamental approach to work allocation, the last phase of planning is the organisation of duty rotas if some system of shift allocation is required.

Many readers will be adept at the practical chore of making duty rotas, but for those with no experience we have produced a logical method of approaching this at the end of this chapter. In making such allocations, account must be taken of several often conflicting factors, such as balance of qualified staff to learners, stage of training of learners, preferences for work hours, balance out unpopular shift allocations, the basic routine for each shift and the proximity of other wards to provide temporary cover for meal breaks, and the availability of relief staff from a 'Bank'.

PROJECT PLANNING

We have concentrated on 'capacity planning' and 'process planning' which are relevant to organising the routines of a unit and scheduling the allocation of staff. There are other tasks which fall to senior nurses, involving the planning of 'one-off' events, such as new training programmes, different treatments, installing new equipment or moving part of a unit. There are several well-established techniques which can be employed in such 'project planning'. As with approaches to routine planning this is basically consolidated common sense, often practised automatically by experienced staff. The emphasis again is on a logical step-by-step method:

1. Define the aims of the project to be planned.

2. Describe the tasks and activities needed to achieve the purpose.
3. Link these into a reasonably logical sequence.
4. Define the resources needed (people, equipment, materials).
5. Allocate time-scales, starting from a predetermined 'end date' and working back, or working forward to an estimated end.
6. Arrange for progress to be monitored.
7. Make some contingency plan.

In complex projects the initial definition of tasks and activities will be essential to ultimate success; again, a 'systems' outlook is relevant. In the 'project' aimed at developing the community health services needed by long-stay patients being discharged from hospital, there is a need to consider also the problems of advice on housing, welfare and other rights, and the provision of day care activities.

Steps 3, 4 and 5 are clearly capable of many different interpretations. One sequence will require more staff to give an earlier completion. Fewer staff will demand a different sequence and a later 'end date'.

One technique for drawing all these steps into one planning document is called 'key events planning'. This is useful for arranging major aspects of work-load in a section for weeks or months ahead, as well as for sorting out one-off projects. The first step is to list all the tasks and activities that are necessary to complete the project. As it is essential to take account of all the tasks involved, it is useful to consult with others at this stage of planninq. This will ensure that nothing is missed. These events can then be written into a time planning sheet, showing exactly when they should occur. Then the processes which have to be completed to achieve these activities can be identified — reading agendas, collecting figures from staff, reading reports, preparing talks, arranging rooms, etc. — and times or dates for undertaking and completing these can be slotted into the time plan.

A variation of this is 'milestone planning', which involves a similar need to specify the key events, but instead of allocating all the

Key events plan			
Issue	Date	Prepared by	Issued to
Dates	Key events		Other events
April 3	Draft programme		Possible speakers found Possible venues
April 6	Programme agreed Speakers agreed		
April 10	Speakers fixed		Audio visual aids Conference papers
April 12	Venue costed and booked		

Milestone plan		
Milestone dates (week-end)	Planned status	
	Main activities	Other activities
April 15	Programme Programme fixed	Content; speakers; venue
April 22	Fee fixed	Printing quotes, speakers' fees, budget approved

Fig. 5.2 Key events and milestone planning.

supporting activities a particular place in the schedule, there is a simple need to predict how many will be completed by the end of each week/day before the final completion time. This acts as a means of checking progress and assessing work priorities when there is an overload.

Another widely used planning technique is the 'Bar chart' or 'Gantt chart'. In this, personal work-load, unit work-load or individual projects can be divided into specific activities and an estimate of the time required to complete each. These are displayed visually by drawing a line across the time and date of each activity in chronological order. Thus routine work can be controlled, or projects given an overall time scale.

At this stage a plan consists of a list of activities linked in some chronological sequence. This might be sufficient to ensure the smooth execution of a project. As manager you know what activities have to be carried out. You can simply direct available staff to undertake the appropriate tasks. If there is a shortage of staff, either try to obtain more, use overtime working, try to speed things up, rearrange your sequence or put the completion date back.

In more complex situations, or where the planning manager is not able to directly supervise the implementation of the plan, a more detailed 'scheduling' will be needed, indicating who is responsible for each activity and estimating the staffing and equipment resources needed.

It is possible to allocate key events to members of the nursing team, indicating when the tasks should be started and completed. It is useful to show the next stage of the sequence and who is responsible, so that if one individual task is delayed the person responsible can approach the next person involved to find ways of coping with the problem. An indication of the most significant tasks can also be given on the schedule.

In project planning, as in planning routine work, the main problems arise in the scheduling stage. The logical approach suggests four basic questions:

1. What separate skills/staff and equipment are required for each activity?
2. When will this staff and equipment be required and for how long?
3. How do these requirements compare with easily available staff and equipment?
4. How can the plan be modified if there is a shortfall of staff or equipment?

One way to illustrate such resource problems revealed in question 4 is the use of a 'histogram'. This is a simple graph with the number of staff or items of equipment on one axis and the days of a week (in routine work planning) or days/weeks from the start date (for project planning) on the other. This graph can then be made to show the peak demand and points where demand exceeds supply. This analysis can then be used to make changes in the sequence of activities so that there are fewer peaks and troughs (Resource smoothing, see Fig. 5.3).

NETWORK PLANNING

Bar chart techniques become too cumbersome for complex project planning involving many people and many activities. Techniques of network planning have been developed for use in these situations, which enable a plan to establish the exact relationship between many activities on a relatively simple diagram.

The first step is to take the list of tasks and make a note beside those which depend on the completion of another task before they can commence (constraints).

Select from the list all activities which have an independent start — they do not have to wait for anything else to happen — and draw circles for each as shown in the illustration in Figure 5.4. These circles are called 'nodes'.

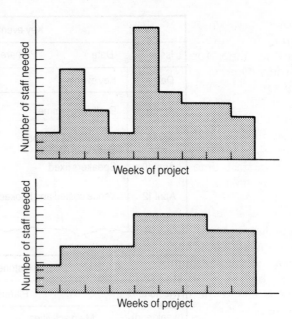

Fig. 5.3 Resource smoothing. The graph above shows unacceptable peaks of labour demand which requires replanning of project activities shown in the graph below.

The next steps involve adding activities which follow each other, joining those together which must be completed before another activity can start (step 2 in Fig. 5.4). In some activities there will be a delay factor as well (printing quotations requested but wait until printer replies) which are shown on the diagram by adding a symbol x (step 3). The progress of a project is plotted on the network by joining further activities and adding the subsequent activity lines to them (step 4); this continues until the project is complete (step 5). The normal convention in presenting networks is to show the conclusion of an activity (termed an 'event') as a small circle by redrawing the network as shown in step 6.

The network will need to show more information to make it of greater use than a bar chart, such as the times involved for each activity and the resources scheduled. From the time-scale, estimates of each activity are added under the lines at the appropriate point on the diagram (step 7), either in hours, weeks etc., depending on the nature of the project. The nodes are also used to record extra time information — earliest possible starting time for an activity (bottom left corner) by adding time figures preceding it on the same line (step 8). On the final node this figure should also be entered in the lower right corner space. Working backwards along every line the right hand corner can be filled with a figure obtained from subtracting the earliest start time (bottom left corner) from the time taken by the preceding activity (step 9). This shows the latest time each activity must be started for the whole network plan to progress.

Following the line through the diagram between the two numbers will trace the activities which have to start and finish on target. This is called the critical path, thus the technique is also called critical path analysis (CPA). The network can be completed by adding schedules which indicate the names of people responsible for each activity (step 10).

This account of the network planning technique has been greatly simplified and gives a brief appreciation only. If a nurse manager becomes involved in a major project that requires such detailed planning it will be useful to make a more careful study of the technique.

PROJECT COSTING

When systematic planning is employed for new projects, it may have an additional use in providing an estimate of the costs involved, which can be used to justify the project and to provide a means of cost control as a project progresses. Thus each activity will need to be analysed in detail to assess the necessary expenditures to complete it. A costing matrix can be drawn up of the activities, which might have to be supported with greater detailed workings of the costs identified.

In producing an estimate of a project cost, it is usual to distinguish between direct expenses and indirect expenses. Direct materials are those which become part of the item being made (paint, wood, etc. to renovate a room); direct labour costs are the wages paid to workers who change the state of the raw materials (maintenance staff, outside subcontractors); direct expenses are other items incurred which are directly attributable to the project (special drawings, hire of equipment, travel). In more detailed costing systems there will also be indirect costs from supervision of project workers, use of power, lighting, depreciation of existing equipment, etc.

In accounting for costs of major projects it may be necessary to distinguish between capital items which are regarded as being assets for an organisation for several years (new buildings, major equipment), and expense items which are only assets in the year they are purchased (maintenance, training, travel).

In commercial organisations, in seeking to justify expenditure of a project an additional consideration is 'cash flow'. This is a comparison of expected revenue to be earned as a direct result of the costs incurred and set against the time that committed costs must be paid. Within the NHS some authorities run cash earning ventures which must be subject to such analysis of cash flow. In deciding to open a shop within a hospital the total cost of building, stocking and staffing will be compared with the forecast income from sales to justify the investment of funds.

Greater detail of the financial management practices applied in the NHS are given in Chapter 21; at this stage it is only necessary for a nurse manager to appreciate that any project that involves expenditure should have properly estimated costings and a budget allocation.

Advice on how projects should be costed in a particular health authority can be obtained from more senior managers or the finance staff.

PLANNING EQUIPMENT

A wide range of products are available to assist managers with planning and organisational tasks. Most readers will be familiar

STEP 1   Identify the separate activities and those dependent on others.

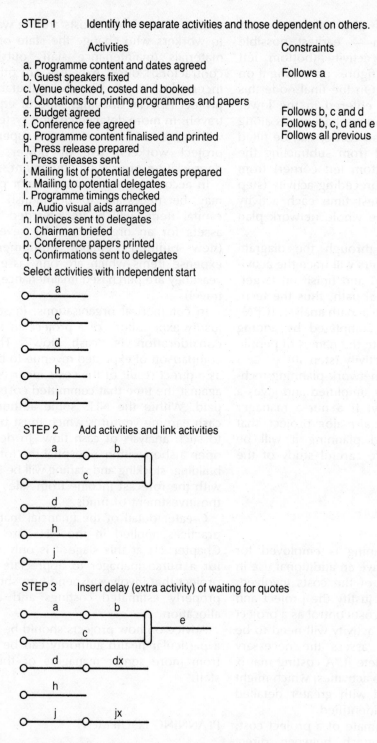

Activities	Constraints
a. Programme content and dates agreed	
b. Guest speakers fixed	Follows a
c. Venue checked, costed and booked	
d. Quotations for printing programmes and papers	
e. Budget agreed	Follows b, c and d
f. Conference fee agreed	Follows b, c, d and e
g. Programme content finalised and printed	Follows all previous
h. Press release prepared	
i. Press releases sent	
j. Mailing list of potential delegates prepared	
k. Mailing to potential delegates	
l. Programme timings checked	
m. Audio visual aids arranged	
n. Invoices sent to delegates	
o. Chairman briefed	
p. Conference papers printed	
q. Confirmations sent to delegates	

Select activities with independent start

STEP 2   Add activities and link activities

STEP 3   Insert delay (extra activity) of waiting for quotes

Fig. 5.4 Network planning. Planning a conference for professional staff.

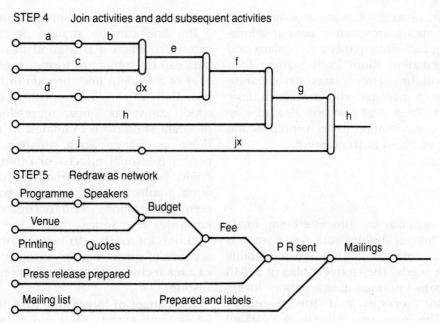

STEP 4 Join activities and add subsequent activities

STEP 5 Redraw as network

Fig. 5.4 (cont'd)

with them but we include a brief description of the most widely used equipment.

Year planners

Wall charts are available which can be used to display key events and activities of a year. Markers can be removable strips in symbols so that these can be easily updated.

Bar chart displays

There are several systems for displaying planning information and information about use of resources. There are basic grids with activities or resources down one side and the time scale across the top. Information can be displayed using card strips, magnetic strips, plastic pins and strips, or slide strips depending on the material of the board and the system design. Another widely used system involves the use of 'T cards', which can contain information about projects, materials, resources, inserted into a board so that only the top bearing an appropriate title is visible.

The use of micro- and mini-computers with

desk top visual display units means that many of these physical systems will become obsolete.

Computers are used in many organisations to assist with project planning and planning of use of resources or, in manufacturing, for production planning. The managers or planners still have to provide information concerning the particular events to be planned; the computer system then evolves a logical plan based on the optimum sequence of activities, and smooths the use of resources to meet time-scales and key events.

There is a separate chapter on computer application with health care (Ch. 22).

We are concerned with the planning process and planning techniques that are of practical significance to nurse managers in the discharge of their routine duties and in contributing efficiently to the future developments of their health care specialisation.

At unit and ward levels there is a need for efficiency in planning for patient care. Such activities, whether undertaken at health authority, or at ward, or at individual patient level, depend on making assumptions about future demand for services. A ward manager with knowledge about prospective patient admissions, using individual patient care plans and having information about likely staffing fluctuations, will be better placed to organise services than a manager who lacks such basic information. Thus it is relevant also to give some brief consideration to the problems and techniques involved in forecasting.

FORECASTING

Every plan depends on forecasts being made about the future. A duty rota for a ward is based on assumptions about staff availability and patient needs. The strategic plan of a RHA relies on many informed guesses about future demand for services and the resources required. The Resources Allocation Working Party (RAWP) recommended a formula for equal distribution of funds across the NHS which depends on forecasts of such factors as mortality, population and mobility (see Ch. 21).

Forecasting at corporate level is an activity requiring considerable amounts of data and the use of relevant quantitative techniques which relate cause and effect in a calculatable way. Sophisticated statistical and operational research methods are mainly the province of specialised staff, but it is essential for practical nurse managers to have some basic appreciation, as well as being aware of the uses and limitations of these techniques.

Forecasting is based on analysis of what has happened in the past and by 'extrapolation' to predict probable future trends. Data must be adequate and representative of a situation, and capable of being analysed. Predictions are made from the study of quantitative measures such as the number of emergency admissions or the number of X-rays over a particular period. Information is plotted on a graph, a trend forecast made from drawing a line which fits past data as nearly as possible to the present. This line is an attempt to smooth out short-term variations to find the average direction of the line and therefore the direction of a trend. This line is extended (extrapolated) to

predict the trend direction in future.

The line can be straight or curved. The extent to which it is a good fit with historic data can be subject to further analysis. In the case of a straight line the sum of the squared deviations of the line from the data points is used, known as 'linear regression'. Clearly, the data should be examined to test predictions, as changes in a situation during the period (seasonal effects) or other influences could suggest an alternative extrapolation. Such graphs of movements of patient treatments, operations, bed occupancy etc. are known as time series.

Other approaches to forecasting take more account of recent figures, using adaptive forecasting techniques such as exponential forecasting.

The danger of forecasting from trends, even when subjected to careful quantitative processing, is that it assumes things will continue as in the past, but in practice changes can arise. Thus shorter-term forecasting and short-term planning have greater reliability. It is essential to consider whether any anticipated events should be taken into account in making predictions.

Nurse managers wishing to undertake forecasting have two sources of data available within their unit, or their hospital:

1. Information which is collected as part of hospital routine for administration and control purposes (admissions and discharge statistics, hours worked, staff employed, etc.)
2. Information which needs to be collected for the specific purpose.

Before collecting data it is essential to decide what detail is needed (patients admitted — by consultant, by diagnosis, previous history, etc.). If the detail required would be too much to handle, a smaller sample of the whole would be used. It is necessary to consider how data is to be checked for bias and errors, as many routine statistics are of suspect reliability.

Information considered useful in forecasting or other decision-making must be processed and interpreted. A common way of looking at data in a time series is to calculate averages. In an emergency unit, from statistics collected over 25 weeks, showing the number of admissions each day, it is easy to find average (or mean) admissions per week (total ÷25), and averages for specific days each week.

Other common ways of interpreting such data is to calculate the median (the value of the scale measure such that half the observations are greater than it and half smaller). This is found by placing, say, the number of X-ray examinations each day for 100 days on a list from the highest to the least, the 50th number giving the median, and the number in the series that occurs most frequently is the 'mode'.

A number of other techniques for presentation and analysis of quantitative data are useful for managers in planning and decision-making. As many readers will be familiar with these techniques, which are not restricted in use to forecasting, we have included further references at the end of Chapter 6.

SYSTEMS PLANNING

There is a danger in using the techniques of 'scientific management' of concentrating on the mechanistic aspects of work and so losing sight of the larger problems. The beginning and end of planning should consider the total 'system' — the complex grouping of human beings and equipment that joins together to achieve a goal or goals.

A single hospital ward is a system with inputs and outputs; it has feedback mechanisms to inform those in charge what changes need to be made with the inputs to achieve desired results. It is an 'open' system in that it is influenced by the rest of the hospital. In turn a hospital is an open system affected by its health authority and the community it serves. Thus, changing one aspect (increasing number of cardiac operations) will have repercussions on other parts of the system (increased medical records, more drugs needed, etc.). Thus a 'systems' view of planning should try to understand how changing one aspect of an existing situation will impact on other aspects.

There are examples of change in health care policy which may have excellent justification but had unfortunate side-effects in other parts of the system. In deciding to release patients from residential treatment in psychiatric hospitals, some districts have found increases in admissions to emergency units of individuals who have been unable to cope back in the community. This has the effect of increasing pressure on beds for patients admitted from 'normal' emergency, yet the health authority were unwilling to provide more emergency resources.

Observing the problem of outpatients having to wait excessively long for an appointment, a health authority might increase resources to have more patients seen per week. If the same proportion of patients requiring further treatment remains constant, however, this change will simply increase the waiting time for inpatient admission, unless further changes are made (increase doctors' availability, more beds, patients' shorter stay in hospital, etc.), but these again will have further consequences in the total system.

Reducing the length of stay in hospital for patients undergoing surgery is claimed to be more efficient as the number of cases treated increases. Some medical authorities have expressed concern, however, that this increases the work load of GPs or increases the rate at which recently discharged patients have to be readmitted.

At ward or unit level it is advisable for nurse managers to adopt a 'systems view' when contemplating change or making decisions. They should consider the possible repercussions in a broad context.

THE ADVANTAGES OF PLANNING

To many experienced sisters or senior nurses some of the techniques we have described will seem unnecessary and too laborious for use in their normal work. Planning will be needed by them, but this will not be committed to paper as their detailed understanding of work tasks, time these should take, staff availability and task priorities will allow much planning to be done 'in the head' and continually modified in the light of practical experience. Where a major project is involved, where there are continuous shortages of resources or where the intuitive approach is not effective, the more disciplined methods of the professional planners may be useful.

A newly promoted nurse manager can also use systematic planning and resource allocation to advantage, as these can facilitate a systematic review of work routines and the possible introduction of new schemes.

Systematic planning will, in addition, give a manager a fundamental tool of the trade — control. A clear understanding of what is supposed to be happening, who is responsible and what the specific targets are, will mean a manager is able to check actual progress against planned achievement, and so take any necessary corrective action.

One obvious danger emerging from a concern with planning and control, however, is that it can lead to resentment and reduced co-operation from staff. This is especially risky for a newly appointed manager who has not established a satisfactory relationship with staff. An essential part of the planning process, therefore, is proper consultation and discussion with staff before plans are made, as well as at the point when a first draft has been made. Not only will this lead to improved staff co-operation but it will mean that staff can introduce practical points and problems that a manager may overlook, thus improving the quality of plans as well. Indeed there are many examples where staff have undertaken to replan work rotas themselves and presented the final outcome to management for approval, as well as examples where professional planners have failed to implement plans because of opposition of staff.

It is also likely that some nurses will regard the prospect of applying these planning processes which have been developed in manufacturing industry, and other techniques of so called 'scientific management' with some scepticism. This is the antithesis of what nursing should be about. The aim of a production planner is to minimise costs and maximise output — that is not the same as caring for sick people. Agreed, but the aim of a nurse manager should be to use staff, materials and equipment in order to serve patient needs in an efficient as well as a caring way. To this end, some useful lessons can be drawn from factory management and work study which can advance the cause of nursing care.

It is important for nurses to be aware of management techniques that are employed by specialists and 'efficiency' experts, so that they can make use of these techniques when appropriate.

METHOD STUDY

Method study is the application of techniques designed to record, by means of charts and diagrams, exactly what is achieved, and challenging, in a logical and systematic manner, why it is being achieved in that way. It is intended that a more effective method can be developed and introduced. These techniques are flexible in that they can be used for a number of different purposes depending on the circumstances, even though the principles and systems for recording are common. The objectives of method study are:

1. To improve the working process
2. To improve the layout of departments or whole buildings
3. To improve the layout of a work area
4. To reduce staff fatigue and improve working conditions
5. To increase equipment utilisation
6. To provide a more effective use of manpower
7. To improve, where possible, 'product design'.

The techiques used to study an existing method of working are those of careful observation, systematic recording on diagrams or charts, and critically questioning each part of the established method. Each of these techniques and the need for critical evaluation should be useful for nurses and nurse managers.

Diagrams and charts

Making a simple diagram can be a useful aid for nurses in planning, both to evaluate the logic in a sequence of work activities, and in displaying a process plan or the schedule of work allocation. From the written list of activities in one process a simple sequence diagram can be made. This consists of using five basic symbols which are linked together to show the flow of a particular process (see Fig. 5.5).

The simplest diagram to produce is an outline process chart which mainly requires the operation and inspection symbols. This is useful in examining the present sequence of activities in a process depicting points where materials or equipment enter. The purpose is to define the best sequence, or to find improvements in the present process (see Fig. 5.6).

Flow process chart

The outline process presents an overall picture of the process. It is often necessary and desirable to go into much greater depth and look at a specific activity rather than the whole process — this is achieved by means of a flow process chart.

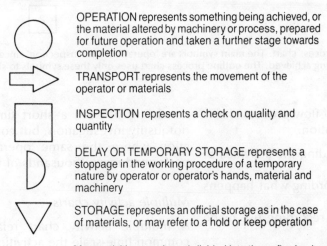

OPERATION represents something being achieved, or the material altered by machinery or process, prepared for future operation and taken a further stage towards completion

TRANSPORT represents the movement of the operator or materials

INSPECTION represents a check on quality and quantity

DELAY OR TEMPORARY STORAGE represents a stoppage in the working procedure of a temporary nature by operator or operator's hands, material and machinery

STORAGE represents an official storage as in the case of materials, or may refer to a hold or keep operation

Most activities may be subdivided into these five basic categories. It may, however, be necessary to combine the symbols if two activities are being performed simultaneously.

For example if an operation was being carried out in conjunction with an inspection then the symbol would be shown thus:-

It is sometimes difficult to decipher which symbol would best represent a particular activity under observation. In these cases consistency is the main requirement, providing the observer is clear as to his choice of symbols.

Fig. 5.5 The ASME symbols. (Developed by the American Society of Mechanical Engineers and known as ASME symbols.)

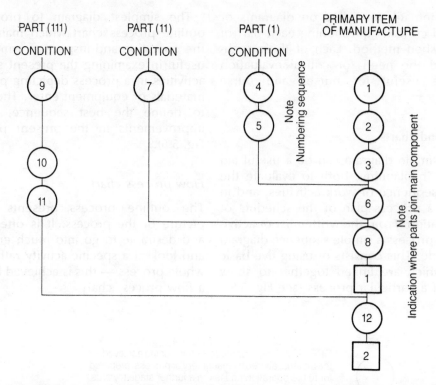

Fig. 5.6 Outline or operation process chart. The main symbols are 'operation' and 'inspection' since these represent activities where something is being achieved. The outline process chart uses only these symbols to show the sequence

There are three types of flow process charts depending on the application.

1. A person type — recording the activities of an individual worker
2. A material type — recording what happens to the material
3. An equipment type — recording use made of the equipment.

All five ASME symbols are used. In addition, it is useful to record the standard time against relevant symbols when known and to record the distances travelled against the relevant transports.

Figure 5.7 shows a flow process chart of a man filling two cans of paraffin from a self-service dispenser. The sequence of activities follows the instructions given on many of these types of machine. The pattern of events seems logical and achieves the objective, but is it necessarily the best method? If the task is performed only once a week, an operation consisting of such a short time-cycle would not justify investigation, but consider the situation where the same operation is being performed many thousands of times a week.

Multiple activity charts

A multiple activity chart relates against a common time-scale the activities of more than one 'operator' or 'machine' or 'operators' and 'machines'.

Taking the same example of a man filling cans with paraffin we have a relationship of one operator with one machine. In this particular case it may prove more advantageous to use a multiple activity chart on which to record, in order that the periods of ineffective time are more clearly shown.

By rearranging the sequence in which the task is performed, the ineffective time of either the machine or the operator will be reduced and thereby increase the utilisation

OPERATION: Filling two cans with paraffin from a self-service dispenser (0.80 gallon per can)

CHART BEGINS: MAN WITH TWO EMPTY CANS AT DISPENSER

PRESENT METHOD

Time	Symbol	Description
(0.04)	①	Place aside 1 empty can to ground
(0.15)	②	Remove lid from remaining can (retaining lid in palm of hand), place hose of dispenser into can and position can to machine
(0.08)	③	Procure coin from pocket and place in coin slot to start pump
(0.27)	D1	Wait for machine to pump 0.80 gallon into glass bowl
(0.06)	④	Operate lever to fill can
(0.29)	D2	Wait for can to be filled
(0.12)	⑤	Remove filled can and replace lid
(0.06)	⑥	Place aside filled can to ground and pick up empty can
(0.15)	⑦	Remove lid from 2nd can (retaining lid in palm of hand), place hose of dispenser into can and position can to machine
(0.08)	⑧	Procure coin from pocket and place in coin slot to start pump
(0.27)	D3	Wait for machine to pump 0.80 gallon into glass bowl
(0.06)	⑨	Operate lever to fill can
(0.29)	D4	Wait for can to be filled
(0.12)	⑩	Remove filled can and replace lid
(0.05)	⑪	Pick up 1st can from ground (retaining 2nd can)

Note that since these activities are a repeat it is possible to insert a comment into the chart to avoid unnecessary charting. The numbering sequence must be continued.

Chart finishes: Man with 2 full cans at dispenser

SUMMARY

Operations	11	Storages	0
Inspections	0	Delays	4
Transports	0	Total time 2.09 std mins	

Fig. 5.7 Flow process chart (man type).

of either the machine or the operator, or both.

Summary

Cycle time	Man	2.09 min	Idle	Man	0.97 min
	Machine	2.09 min		Machine	1.12 min
Working	Man	1.12 min	% Utilisation	Man	53.6 %
	Machine	0.97 min		Machine	46.4 %

Working periods are shaded or coloured to emphasise the idle time of the operator and the machine. The summary gives the total periods of working, non-working and

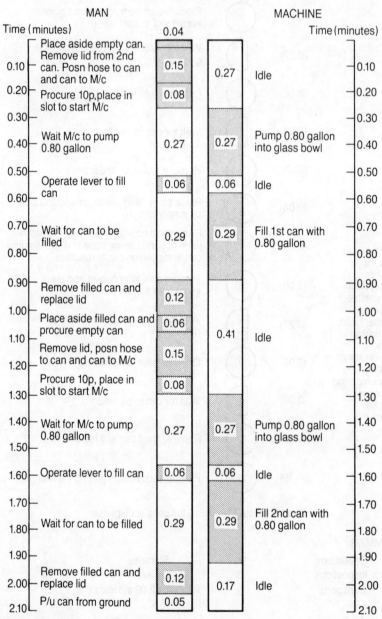

Fig. 5.8 Multiple activity chart (man–machine process chart).

percentage utilisation, and indicates the scope for improvement.

An accurate means of work measurement was used to establish the times indicated: it is possible to use an ordinary clock or wrist-watch to obtain times depending on the circumstances.

This example of multiple activity chart or man/machine chart, as this particular one is sometimes known, shows only two related functions in a process. Other charts involving a team of workers or an operator and several machines are built up in much the same way. Usually only one time-scale is used with each function charted separately, yet still in relation to the others.

Diagrams for planning layouts

Part of a logical approach to the initial planning of a unit, or to investigate possible improvements in an existing set-up involves a critical review of possible layouts for equipment. Professional planning staff make use of a variety of diagrams to assist in these tasks.

The flow diagram is a simple means of showing the movement of material or a worker against a drawing of the work place: this is not necessarily to scale. This can be shown to great advantage in conjunction with a flow process chart to give a more concise picture of man or material movements.

The three-dimensional diagram is a development of the flow diagram; it is useful in illustrating the flow of materials or movement of operators over a number of different working levels.

Drawings are not necessarily to scale, but are designed to give a clearer understanding and are used as a 'back-up' to the flow process chart.

Another diagram used for establishing the movement of worker and materials is the string diagram.

It is necessary to start with a scale drawing of the working area, giving the exact positions of all the relevant machines, benches, racks, stores etc.

The drawing is placed on a board suitable

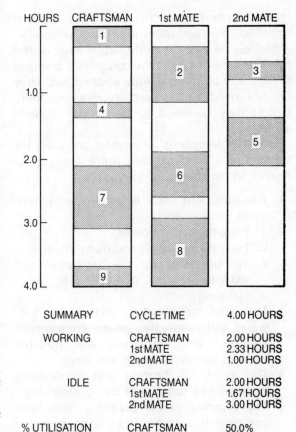

SUMMARY	CYCLE TIME	4.00 HOURS
WORKING	CRAFTSMAN	2.00 HOURS
	1st MATE	2.33 HOURS
	2nd MATE	1.00 HOURS
IDLE	CRAFTSMAN	2.00 HOURS
	1st MATE	1.67 HOURS
	2nd MATE	3.00 HOURS
% UTILISATION	CRAFTSMAN	50.0%
	1st MATE	58.3%
	2nd MATE	25.0%

Fig. 5.9 Multiple activity chart (team of workers).

for receiving pins. A fine string or thread is used to depict the movements of the man or materials about the workplace and is supported by pins at the stopping and turning points.

When re-organising the layout of a department it is useful to prepare a scale drawing of the department showing the main walls, doorways and girders. Templates are made to scale of the machines and equipment, being careful to allow for equipment movement and work.

Models are used in the same way as templates except that scale replicas of machines, equipment, etc. are made instead of two-dimensional cut-outs. Similarly a scale model of the unit or department is made showing walls and roof supports. To this 'shell' is added the route of essential services (gas, water and electricity), heating, pipes and radiators, plus any other important factors.

Models do give the added advantage of the third dimension and allow proposed changes in layout to be more readily understood. They do not need to be exact replicas to finite detail; they do need to be proportionately accurate.

Whether templates or models are used for laying out a working area there are certain factors which should be considered:

1. That sufficient space is left around equipment to allow for:
   a. Equipment movement
   b. Essential servicing and maintenance
   c. Working area for the 'operator' and work in progress, materials, etc.
   d. Gangways
2. The need for essential services, i.e. gas, water and electricity, steam, compressed air, etc., and that these are available without too much additional cost
3. The need for heating and ventilation, extraction of fumes and air conditioning
4. The *accuracy* of the drawings, templates and models — error can be *very* expensive
5. The positioning of stauntions, manhole covers, etc.
6. The safety of personnel
7. The size of doorways and openings in relation to equipment to be moved
8. The need for additional lighting
9. The need for new spaces and equipment
10. The weight of equipment and floor loading

The purpose in using these quite elaborate techniques as an aid to planning is to find improvements to efficiency of working. Thus the two basic questions 'What is achieved?' and 'Is it really necessary?' should be used together with supplementary questions 'How, where, when and by whom else could an activity or sequence be planned to achieve the purpose?'

Examining the present process in a critical way means it is possible to find ways of reducing 'down time' — times when equipment or staff are being underutilised. A nurse manager can adopt a similar critical outlook to question established practice, but also taking into account the realities of nursing care and protection of professional standards.

In one comparison of the organisation of an intensive care unit in Zurich University Hospital and that current in the UK at the time (Gibson, 1986) it was found that the Swiss practice had advantages. 'The outstanding difference is their more efficient use of nurse manpower, made possible by the deployment of nurses according to patients' nurse dependency . . . the absence of ritualistic timing of recording observations.'

It appears that the system was more efficient in the use of ITU nurses but maintained standards as it enabled 'the maximum number of patients to receive cardiac surgery and the standards of care and mortality rates have not suffered as a result.'

Planning duty rotas

One of the most time-consuming tasks for the average ward sister is planning the duty rota for staff. It takes time to master the art of planning at this level, as there are many points to take into account. Hospitals generally have set duty shifts for nursing staff, so the ward sister has to work within this overall constraint. The shifts are usually 'early' and 'late day' shifts and a night shift. There are several advantages to hospital administration in such a pattern of working, notably that hours of work can be easily monitored; with equal shift hours staff can be interchangeable and the organisation of transport and meal breaks is easier.

The main aim at ward level should be to produce balanced duty rotas with adequate cover for days achieved by juggling with early and late shifts. The night duty rota is often planned by the night nurse co-ordinator who plans the night shift for a whole hospital.

A ward sister should attempt to keep a fairly even number and balance of grades throughout the day, concentrating more staff to weekdays. At weekends the level of ward activity is reduced thus taking less staff. In undertaking the detailed planning to achieve this overall aim there are several factors to be assessed:

1. The number of staff available, including learners. The fact that the actual allocation of learners to a ward can vary considerably, as does the stage they have reached in their training, can produce several planning problems. With the modular system of training ward sisters may find the majority of learners are in their first year or have come directly from an introductory block. These nurses require much more direct supervision than learners in the third year.
2. The grade mix within the staff. For a general ward, depending on bed allocation, there will be a mix of sisters, staff nurses, enrolled nurses, nursing auxiliaries and learner nurses (students and pupils).
3. The time when staff are away from the ward for various reasons and are generally not replaced, i.e annual leave, study leave, long-term sickness, maternity leave.
4. The need to give days off for individual staff so that they get the longest break, if possible by allocating an early shift before and a late shift afterwards.
5. The need to take account of the duty requests from staff. The expectation today is that the demands of nurses' domestic and social commitments should be considered whenever possible.
6. The learner nurses' next allocations have to be considered; if they are on night duty next they should be given time off beforehand.
7. The need to ensure that each nurse has an even mixture of late and early shifts without too many of the same in a row.
8. The need to match staff grades to patient needs and ward activities.

It would be an advantage for ward sisters to have greater flexibility in planning duty rotas instead of having to conform to the rigid hospital structures irrespective of the particular areas of care. An examination of the typical pattern of work over a 24 hour period and over each day of the week would indicate the optimum level of staff required for specific wards/units. Nurses' attitudes towards greater flexibility are changing, which helps to reduce the peaks and troughs of demand on a ward and avoids the practice of waking patients early in the morning for a 9 am ward round.

The hospital's shift system has been subject to review to assess whether it is efficient, particularly the need for overlap of staff between early and late day shift. The justification for this arrangement is that it allows for many important activities to be carried out without reducing care given to patients. The overlap enables nurses to give and receive verbal reports on patient care, have in-service teaching and training sessions, attend a variety of meetings and have a meal break. Another recent development that has an influence on planning rotas is the organisation of nursing to give individualised patient care.

There is now increasing use of computers in hospitals to assist nurse managers in planning duty rotas. This trend should mean that a better match is achieved between staff resources and work-load while saving ward sisters considerable time.

REFERENCES

Applin L 1984 Shift systems. Nursing Times, May
DHSS 1983 Operational research service. Nurse manpower planning and techniques. HMSO, London
Gibson S 1986 Swiss precision. Nursing Times, March 26th
Grant N 1979 Time to care. RCN, London
Long D 1986 Critical Path Analysis, Hodder and Stoughton Sevenoaks
Moore P 1986 Basic operational research. Pitman, London
Pearson A 1983 The clinical nursing unit. William Heinemann, London
Pembrey S 1980 The ward sister: The key to nursing. RCN, London
Perry E 1978 Ward management and teaching, Bailliere Tindall, London

What to monitor

How to monitor

Control by exception

Decision-making

6
Monitoring and controlling

The responsibility of exercising control over the work of more junior staff can present a serious dilemma. There is a need for all senior nurses to demonstrate to their immediate seniors, consultants and general managers that they are in command of their unit. At the same time it is essential that their own staff feel that they are given support and informed guidance. There is a danger that a ward sister, from a desire to exercise tight control, will be seen by staff as interfering and showing no trust in them. Yet if the sister tries a freer approach, she may be regarded by other managers as lacking necessary discipline.

A similar dilemma can be present in the more senior levels of a nursing hierarchy. Here control of a patient care service should be exercised in a more remote style through the reporting relationship with first-line supervision and middle managers.

From a desire to be sure that everything is done properly, however, there is a temptation to go directly onto wards, by-passing and undermining ward level supervision. It is not possible to achieve total management control in the sense of being able to direct and command others to behave exactly as management intends. Only totalitarian political regimes, or totally authoritarian management, would seek to dominate the hearts and minds of citizens or staff. In democratic societies and modern organisations it is expected that individuals at all levels will exercise some responsible self-control; it is recognised that individuals should question the decisions of leaders and make a contribution to planning and decision-making.

Managers have no 'divine right' to manage. They are constrained by the policies, procedures, rules and agreements, customs and culture of the organisation in which they are employed. At the most senior level they are inhibited by political, economic and social pressures, by a considerable amount of legislation and by the representation of trades unions and community groups.

In the face of such limitations on the power of management, some managers, especially in lation and by the representation of trade decline the attempt to exercise any authority. They refer problems to higher line management or functional specialists, and wait for a decision which they simply pass on to those concerned.

Clearly, such an abdication by managers at any level is undesirable. Even in centralised bureaucracies all managers need to exercise some control. The main objective of first-line nurse management is to ensure that the appropriate quality of care is provided consistently. As it is undesirable, as well as impossible, to spend every working minute in direct supervision of staff, a decision has to be made on *what* to monitor and *how* to monitor it, as well as how to make effective decisions when things are not working satisfactorily.

WHAT TO MONITOR

Today the concept of 'monitoring' is more applicable than that of 'controlling' and 'commanding'. The aim is to understand what is happening in work, to assess whether targets are being achieved so that timely decisions can be made to get back on course or to modify targets. Thus establishing standards of performance and identifying key result areas will establish 'what' to monitor. Obtaining information from appropriate sources will provide the 'how' of monitoring.

We have given some indication of the means and problems involved in identifying possible key results areas for nurse managers. Broadly, the sources discussed in Chapter 2 were — formal job descriptions; unit procedures and standing orders; agreements within a health care team; health authority indicators of performance and professional codes of conduct. At this point we are concerned with the definition of practical standards for the work of a nursing unit.

Without awareness of key results and agreement on quality requirements, managers are in danger of monitoring the wrong things and relying on subjective judgements. In education, the key result areas should be delivery of appropriate learning to students, yet many schools do not require information which gives an on-going picture of tutor effectiveness in this vital area. The number of hours spent lecturing, the number of students per group, the level of absenteeism might be recorded. The only way a director of studies can find out about teaching quality is if things go seriously wrong, so that students complain or drop out of courses, or finally from poor examination results, when it is too late to rectify the situation.

There are those in medicine and nursing who are sceptical of attempts to apply 'business' management control methods to health care. They contend that as patients are individuals and the progress of treatments and general circumstances vary in different parts of the Health Service, precise measures are unrealistic. The argument can be taken a stage further.

Given the difficulties in agreeing on exact standards in some of the less tangible aspects of patient care, the problem of monitoring key areas and the fact that health care workers are well trained, it is clear that health care management has to rely on the skill and integrity of staff. In a 'professional bureaucracy', control systems should reflect the quality of staff rather than attempt to monitor every detail of performance. If this does apply, it is likely that the emphasis will be directed towards identifying errors and deviations from the standard. Management will only seem interested in the work of staff when things go wrong. An effective control system is one that monitors complete performance. Managers should recognise when things are going well and be prepared to give praise for consistent good performance or for efforts above the norm.

Despite the difficulties in monitoring and control, the increasing emphasis on 'value for money' in health care means that continuous efforts will be made to define standards.

HOW TO MONITOR

The essential requirement for effective monitoring is timely and reliable information from a work-force. Feedback provides the control loop which enables work processes to be regulated. Managers need to identify the information that is likely to be most appropriate in providing the control loop.

The principle of quality control systems, that quality checks should be made at significant moments in a 'production' cycle, is appropriate in all organisations. In manufacturing, the key quality control should be applied on the receipt of raw materials and at each stage where the materials undergo modifications. The aim is to pick out errors early to prevent further work and resources being wasted on faulty items, rather than only inspecting the finished product to reject substandard work. Ward sisters should identify significant points in the work of a ward and the treatment of patients so that control can be applied to prevent serious errors rather than applying it after these have occurred. Similar principles should apply to managing community nursing services.

There are three distinct forms of information required as feedback for management control. These are:

1. Historic: Summary of expenditure provided by a financial officer showing actual costs against budget etc. (see Ch. 21 for a further account of budgeting control). Analysis of bed occupancy. Report on stock levels held, etc.

2. Current: List of absentees on night shift. List of admission to a unit. Current level of bed occupancy. Nursing process plans for each patient etc.
3. Forecast: Off duty rota showing staffing levels for next week. Operations schedules etc.

Information to be of practical use needs to come to managers at an appropriate *time*, which means that the manager needs to know where to find it, so it must be *accessible*, as well as being *reliable* which will mean it is *useful*. Management information (historic, currrent, forecast) is available from four main sources:

1. Records

Statistical returns and summaries giving indication of standards adhered to and resources available. Nurse managers should have readily available records on many items about a unit or speciality such as:

— Staff in post and established level
— Brief personal details of staff (full records held by personnel department)
— Individual staff development plans (see Ch. 19).
— Attendance and absence records
— Changes of medical staff and non-medical staff
— Ward placement for nurses in training
— Training activity records
— Bed reductions/increases
— Patient visits
— Bed occupancy analysis
— Patient admissions/discharges
— Requisitions issued for stores, maintenance etc.
— Incidents on ward/hospital/district
— Budget and expenditure
— Staff meeting minutes
— Management meeting minutes
— Complaints.

In addition to general data concerning the ward it is useful to maintain records which could be used for research, development or forecasting purposes. These may cover treatments given, patient problems, materials used, wastage of materials, infections, use of relief staff, bed occupancy etc. An essential aspect of monitoring is recording the progress of patient treatments by the maintenance of detailed, up-to-date patient records.

2. Reports

Regular reviews of general activities from emergency units/wards/community etc., as well as information on the progress of projects, the outcome of investigation etc., should be provided in the form of verbal or written reports. At ward level there will be the verbal hand-over report between senior shift staff, reports of incidents being written into a ward report book. Sisters will be required to present periodic reports on their ward/patients/cases for health care team or ward sister meetings etc. Senior nurses will be required to summarise information from records and from ward reports for higher management to monitor performance.

3. Observation

Most first-line supervisors adopt a system of regularly 'walking the job' as a way of directly monitoring standards. This can either be at set times (start of shift, mid-shift, just before shift ends) or at random intervals. The aim is to be available with advice which will avoid mistakes and delays, to make spot checks on quality and progress of work, and to deliver praise for good work. Higher ranks of management can also usefully make direct contact with nursing staff, but the intention should be to offer encouragement and show interest, not to undermine the role of first-line managers.

4. Extra information

Feedback to assist managers with control can come from sources outside the immediate section being supervised. Discussions with doctors and with senior nurses in specialised advisory posts will provide information useful for contingency decision-making. Data from personnel, organisation and methods, the finance officer and administrators can be similarly useful. Within each ward or unit there will also be established procedures to be used in emergency situations which include contact with senior nursing managers. Complaints and compliments from patients and relatives are another form of feedback which gives a manager further information on the extent to which quality standards are being maintained. It is possible to seek patient/client reactions in a systematic way by interviews and questionnaires giving measures of their satisfaction with services provided.

This control model might suggest that the main factor in getting things right is management rather than the professional staff who actually work with patients. The purpose of management should be to ensure that staff are conscientious in self-regulation. The provision of checklists which nurses can use to ensure all stages of a procedure are followed, or nurses working in pairs for the issue of drugs on a ward, are methods which encourage self-regulation. This must be a significant feature of effective control.

Controlling vital elements of patient treatment under intensive care is now largely a matter of technology. The aim is to remove or reduce to a non-crucial level the danger of human error. Outside the acute areas, or for more routine matters, control still depends on staff being able to obtain useful control information. With the volume of reports, records and personal observation available, it is important for every manager not only to get information but also to have a reliable filing system. This will mean that essential information can be located quickly. Increasingly, computers will be taking over the tasks of storing, processing, locating and presenting information. Already nursing managers in some health authorities are able to call up details of admissions and operating lists onto the screen of a visual display unit (see Ch. 22).

CONTROL BY EXCEPTION

So far we have suggested a control system that would be applied equally towards all aspects of a unit's work. This is clearly the safest policy. In practice, however, managers find that some staff are more reliable and more skilled than others. They therefore need less close supervision and may be managed with a 'control by exception' style. Agreement is reached about the possible circumstances in which such a subordinate should refer to the manager for advice and what general reporting procedure is appropriate. Under such an arrangement the control system is left more to the discretion of staff members than their immediate supervisor.

In some areas of nurse management such a style of control will be the most appropriate. Where qualified and competent district nurses and health visitors are working in the community, control by exception will generally apply. Similarly in hospital, where junior staff possess considerable knowledge and skill in a particular nursing specialism and have demonstrated reliability, greater autonomy will be granted. In monitoring night sisters it may be appropriate to provide a senior nurse as an 'on call' resource, rather than actively supervising.

DECISION-MAKING

In seeking to analyse management as a specific occupation it is necessary to discuss different aspects in apparent isolation. This is not how managers act in practice. Each day, management work consists of a variety of short-span tasks, the most common of which is talking with other people. To an onlooker this appears to be a somewhat haphazard and disjointed process, nothing like the efficient-sounding formula of establishing objectives, planning, monitoring and controlling etc. In practice an effective manager is still exercising these skills, but has to switch rapidly from one to the other.

At the start of each shift a ward sister may have a brief meeting with the sister from a previous shift and the senior ward staff. This will be an aid in planning to overcome immediate problems threatening the smooth running of the ward. A visit to wards may follow and be part of the monitoring and controlling process. Later, there may be interviews for staff recruitment (developing), a training session (developing) and further planning through a nurse managers' meeting.

However, there are common skills present in every aspect of a manager's work — obtaining information and decision-making — although we shall examine decision-making processes in the context of management control.

For nurse managers in direct line management posts each day will be filled with problems. Not all problems are difficult or unpleasant to deal with; many are routine occurrences which experienced nurses can take in their stride. Inevitably, there will also be circumstances more demanding of decision-making abilities. Some supervisors try to avoid such pressure by referring the problem on to someone else, probably the next most senior manager, but also to more junior staff. If this strategy is not available they prevaricate in the hope that the problem will disappear of its own accord. Clearly, these are not the approaches of a responsible manager.

Everyone who aspires to a management role needs the ability to recognise problems and make effective decisions that fall within their delegated authority. In circumstances where authority is lacking or is unclear, it is still necessary to analyse problems and arrive at possible solutions which can then be referred for ratification by an appropriate senior person.

In practice it is difficult to assess whether a managerial decision is right. There are rarely means available to test objectively whether alternative solutions would have worked out any better, or any worse. At times subjective opinions suggest that a poor decision has been made. The causes are usually:

1. Insufficient information has been obtained on which to base a sound decision.
2. Only an incomplete analysis and understanding of a problem has taken place.
3. There has been too much concern with finding a quick solution to a problem.
4. There has been a tendency to allocate blame to others for causing the problem rather than being concerned with finding a satisfactory solution.
5. Managers have been too emotionally involved, or too close to a problem for rational analysis.
6. There has been a preference to adopt conventional solutions to a problem.

If decisions are based on a process of logical thought and discussion they are more likely to be 'right'. As much of the practice and education of medical professionals is based on the application of scientific method, it should be easy for senior nurses to adopt a similar approach to managerial decision-making. We describe below the preferred method as it can be applied to a practical nurse management problem.

Example

A senior nurse in a general hospital faced difficulties with one of her sisters who was responsible for the operating theatre. The sister had become extremely concerned about the way the registrar arranged lists for operations. She complained continually to the registrar but he took no notice. This made her criticisms even more outspoken: so much so that the registrar complained to the senior nurse that she 'bombarded' him whenever they came into contact. The sister complained to the senior nurse about the registrar's rudeness.

A rational approach in this situation was difficult as the senior nurse was both emotionally involved and inhibited by the status of the registrar. A logical sequence in tackling it was as relevant to this problem as to any other. The stages in rational problem-solving can involve a number of questions to be asked by the decision taker:

1. What is the problem about? There are often two or three problems interwoven which need to be separated. In this case, the sister's manner in approaching the problem, the actual difficulties in the preparation of lists and the registrar's attitude need separate consideration.
2. Whose problem is it? (Does the senior nurse really have to solve it? What authority does she have?)
3. Is there any more information required before a decision can be made? (Why does the Registrar adopt his approach? What are the practical problems?)
4. Are there any organisational rules, procedures, customs or future developments that have any bearing on this problem? (Have previous discussions been held with the registrar? Is the sister likely to continue in the theatre?)
5. What exactly is the problem to be solved? (Many people can complain about the difficulties of a situation but this does not always give a positive expression of the problem. In this case the senior nurse appeared to have two problems to resolve — 'How can the sister be encouraged to change her approach to the registrar?' and 'How can the operations list be organised more effectively?')
6. How urgent is the problem? (Does it need immediate attention?)
7. What are some (or all) of the possible approaches/solutions to the problem? (See the Registrar first. See the Sister first. See them together. Move the Sister. Leave things alone etc.)
8. What are the likely outcomes of each possible course of action and what are the merits? (What might be achieved? What are the likely repercussions? What are the net gains? Are precedents likely to be established?)
9. Who should be consulted or informed about this problem? Who should be involved in the decision-making task?

10. Can any possible solutions be checked or tested out before application? (Use trial run, pilot scheme etc.)
11. What follow-up would be needed to ensure that the final decision achieves the purpose? (written agreement, further meetings etc.)
12. What caused the problem in the first place? Can the cause be removed to prevent further problems?
13. What have I/we learned from this experience?

In the problem confronting the senior nurse she decided to talk to the sister first. She endeavoured to separate the two issues of the practical theatre problems and the Sister's manner in trying to resolve them. After a very difficult conversation the sister came to accept that her manner had been inappropriate. The senior nurse had taken full account of the details of her complaints as well. She took up these with the registrar in an equally difficult meeting.

Eventually he agreed that some practical changes could be beneficial in management of the operations list which would meet the main complaints of the sister.

This framework for a logical approach to management problems is based on the most simple but indisputable principle 'think before you act'. There are many decisions which are either made too swiftly or from a fixed point of view which follows on the first solution that comes to mind without full account of the possible repercussions. The list of questions above may seem too elaborate for making decisions on everyday problems in running a hospital ward. Good managers check through the stages quickly as a matter of routine, however. It need not be time consuming in relatively simple circumstances. In complex issues or matters of some significance it is better to take time in order that a sound decision is made.

It is useful in these circumstances to put things down on paper. Simple notes under each step of the logical process can be of great assistance. Listing, in any order, possible solutions to a problem and noting beside each the 'pros' and 'cons' can be similarly useful. Listing activities and sequences can help to identify the best approach to implementing a decision. A form of a simple network can be employed to enable each alternative course of action to be plotted to conclusion. An

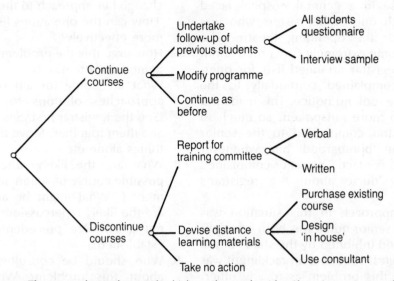

Fig. 6.1 Decision trees. These are a form of network which can be used to identify various courses of action available to resolve a problem. With a simple problem concerning the continuation of a training programme which has been under criticism a tree might be constructed as shown above.

example of such a 'decision tree' is shown in Figure 6.1

In recent years, specialised study of the process of organisation decision-making has developed with several elaborate techniques to assist managers with complex problem-solving. These apply mathematical analysis and models to the complex factors in decisions. It is possible to simulate the circumstances surrounding a decision in order to identify the likely consequences from trends and from alternative courses of action.

These and other quantitative applications have been employed by 'management scientists' in 'operational research' and 'cybernetics'. All follow logical processes in applying mathematical analysis (using linear programming, dynamic programming, game theory and probability theory) to management and organisational problems. The main characteristics of such decision theories are:

1. Construction of a *mathematical model* that satisfies the conditions of the tools to be used and which, at the same time, mirrors the important factors in the management situation to be analysed.
2. Define the *criterion function*, the measures to be used for comparing the relative merits of various possible courses of action.
3. Obtain *empirical estimates* of the numerical parameters in the model that specify the particular, concrete situation to which it is to be applied.
4. Carry through the mathematical processes of finding the course of action to which it is to be applied.

In this scientific approach to decision-making there is an attempt to be logical, but also to adopt a 'systems view' by taking account of many variables in assessing the likely outcome of a particular course. There have been a number of applications of operational research to health care problems, such as an identification of the need for an intensive therapy unit, planning a surgery, and work-load analysis, (Luck et al 1971).

There is a danger in regarding these logical approaches to decision-making as isolated activities where the individual manager acts in a computer-like manner to process data, list possible solutions and simulate outcomes. In reality it is often necessary and usually desirable to involve others at various stages. This should ensure a rigorous discussion to find an accurate definition of a problem, access to more information, more ideas on possible solutions, varied experiences and opinions to consider the practicality of ideas and, most importantly, commitment to the implementation of the final decision. We give a more detailed account of the particular skills needed to lead a small group of staff or managers through a decision-making meeting in the section about communication (Ch. 9).

We have examined an important aspect of effective nurse management, that of being able to monitor the work of a unit to assess whether desired standards are being achieved. This indicates the need to make decisions of varying magnitude and therefore call on the skills of logical decision-making. Thus by knowing what key aspects to monitor, having reliable information to give timely feedback and making considered decisions, nurse managers should be able to exercise control. There are other vital elements in management control, however — that is planning and controlling our own work activities to maximum effect as well as being effective in delegating to others.

REFERENCES

Cooke S, Slack N 1984 Making management decisions. Prentice Hall, New Jersey
Day C 1985 From figures to facts. King's Fund, London
Luck, Luckman, Smith, and Stringer, 1971 Patients, hospitals and operational research. Tavistock, London
Moore P 1986 Basic operational research. Pitman, London
Oates G 1984 Nursing implications of Korner report. Nursing Times, May
Tyrell M 1975 Using numbers for effective health service management. Heinemann, London

7

Controlling your own work by effective time management

An important requirement in seeking to exercise control and influence on the work of others is to be in control of your own work. If you expect others to achieve results it is important to ensure that you get the most out of each day by directing your energies in a purposeful way. Effective managers have to develop appropriate control systems for themselves.

Planning and monitoring the use of time and concentrating this precious resource on the right priorities is essential for nurse managers at every level, especially in circumstances where resources are being reduced but where pressure to deliver a service continues. Even in non-management roles there is often some autonomy in allocating time and an absence of close supervision, which means effective time management is necessary for professional staff as well.

In any senior position it is unlikely that all work tasks will be easily contained within a working day, or a working week. Because an individual is committed to a profession, likes to work hard and is prepared to give more hours than are strictly required by a contract of employment, it does not necessarily mean that this is a symptom of poor time management.

However, it is possible to identify many managers who actually cause greater pressures on themselves than are necessary to fulfil their role objectives in a responsible manner. It is important for all managers to be aware of the symptoms, the likely causes and the possible solutions to time management problems.

SYMPTOMS OF TIME MANAGEMENT PROBLEMS

The most basic symptom is that of being over busy yet not achieving much in the key results areas of a role. Many managers report that they are haunted by a feeling of always 'running late', of having more and more to do but less and less time to do it in. They tend to go from crisis to crisis so that the job is on top of them instead of being the other way round.

Of course, a certain level of stress as a result of crises is stimulating and is necessary in maintaining an interest in work and in developing fresh skills and knowledge. Perpetual crises, however, lead to unhealthy consequences and inefficient working habits.

There is likely to be a feeling of stress which can lead to poor decision-making and undermine human relationships, both in work and outside. To cope with an unremitting workload, poor time managers often arrive for work early, spend the day hopping from task to task, rarely completing anything satisfactorily despite doing two or more things simultaneously. They work during meal-breaks, after the official end of the day and probably take work away on the expectation of doing some more on a journey or at home. Despite this obvious dedication to work such managers give the impression of being disorganised, are unable to give attention to training and coaching subordinates and are insensitive to the needs of others around them.

CAUSES OF TIME MANAGEMENT PROBLEMS

In seeking to assess the causes of time management problems it is useful to distinguish between those that are rather outside the control of the individual manager and those which are more appropriately attributed to individual style and ineffectiveness.

Unremitting work pressure and continuous crisis management are more commonly associated with sharp end departments in any organisation. Where there is an unpredictable or uneven work-load, where there is a demand to meet strict deadlines and rigid standards, there is likely to be crisis. In hospitals, nurse managers who are responsible for accident and emergency departments may experience this problem. In these circumstances, a senior nurse can be drawn into direct patient care to overcome the crisis, thus pushing administration and management tasks to one side. However competent first-line managers are, it should be recognised that planning and allocating time in a balanced way will be more difficult than in more easily regulated sections.

Similarly, some managers are placed in organisational roles where they have too many direct subordinates to supervise, or have to report to several seniors. In one hospital the director of nursing services had eight nursing officers, four reporting directly and four through an SNO. This structure meant the director was drawn into short-term problems of the four nursing officers (acting down as a SNO), thus making it difficult to maintain a proper long-term perspective.

Time difficulties for middle and junior managers can be created by the attitude of their seniors. If you report to a manager who demands that you have complete and detailed knowledge of the section you supervise, and is likely to call for such information without warning, it is difficult to adopt a 'management by exception' style. There is likely to be duplication of effort and excessive monitoring, thus causing unnecessary work.

Working for a senior who is poorly organised and ineffective at planning her work, will probably mean she dumps tasks on subordinates at short notice, thus disrupting their work schedules.

Although such organisational problems as sharp end management, unbalanced structure, over-zealous or poorly organised senior staff are likely to be a problem anywhere, some nurse managers still cope well whilst others cause themselves unnecessary time management pressures.

The most common self-induced cause is that of poor planning, both in application to the work of a section and to your own work tasks. In some respects this is a self-perpetuating problem. A manager who struggles with the many tasks and problems that arrive at her door will not have time to plan; a manager who does not plan ahead will inevitably tackle the most immediately pressing tasks.

A second managerial weakness that is both a cause and consequence of poor time management is that of ineffective delegation. Ensuring that staff (as well as your colleagues and your bosses) take their fair share of work of the appropriate difficulty, whilst monitoring sufficiently, without interfering, are the basis of effective delegation. (See p. 76 for more detailed discussion.)

After planning and delegation, self-discipline is the key to getting the most out of each day. Some common time-consuming habits which affect even the most senior managers include:

— Putting off difficult or unpleasant tasks
— Starting but failing to finish unpleasant work tasks
— Being easily side-tracked
— Procrastination on necessary decisions
— Poorly organised desk, filing and layouts
— Poor at organising and conducting meetings
— Attending too many meetings
— Talking too much — 'Socialising' in work
— Being too nosey — wishing to be involved in everything
— Not being able to refuse others' requests for help
— Being too visible, too easily accessible.

The most common cause of time slippage in work is being interrupted by others, either in person or on the telephone. Even managers who are careful about planning their day, working on priority tasks and exercising self-restraint are prey to others interrupting them. Not that all interruptions are destructive. Some bring valuable information, or help others to overcome a difficult problem. The ability to rate the likely importance of an interruption and managing your activities so that interruptions are to a minimum are essential.

POSSIBLE SOLUTIONS

A good 'time manager' is one who:

— Seeks to eliminate as far as possible organisational structure problems
— Seeks to manage senior staff as well as colleagues
— Plans her own work as much as possible
— Delegates effectively
— Exercises self-discipline in work
— Exercises control to limit unnecessary interruptions.

Planning work

There are several specially prepared time planning systems for managers. These can be useful but can be easily made by adapting a conventional business diary.

The most important starting point is not owning a time planning system but having a clear view of priorities and the practicability of forward planning.

The job description of 'clinical nurse manager', described on page 11, shows a key responsibility is that of ensuring proper levels of staffing on nights, and a proper structure of nursing care. Problems in these activities will probably take priority at the start and end of each shift. Once overall staffing has been organised, the job holder would probably become involved in discussions of nursing care problems and practices in the orthopaedic unit. There will be inevitable calls for advice from other wards and some crisis to manage. There will be meetings to attend and routine administration to complete. It would be possible for the senior nurse to respond to such pressures and use her diary only to make time for meetings and other requested appointments. This would not be effective time management.

There are other key areas where initiative will be required by the senior nurse. 'Identifying learning needs ... acting as educator and facilitator for all staff on night duty', are tasks requiring a long planning cycle. So the senior nurse should allocate time in her diary over this period, either as milestones by which time all staff learning needs will be assessed, or with specific dates when various interviews and discussions might be arranged to advance the diagnosis of training needs.

Similarly, dates for training periods should be identified in advance which will then allow sub-tasks needed to prepare a session to be planned in sequence over a suitable period.

Thus the elements of time planning systems are to create a list of tasks for each working day which mix long and short-term goals whilst leaving enough space for the immediate and unpredictable. To arrive at such a daily plan it is useful to start with an overview of a year or at least several months ahead, filling in milestones and fixed events (staff appraisal interviews completed June 1st, budget requests required by October 31st, monthly unit meetings etc.), then to create a more detailed plan for the immediate month with appropriate tasks related to these fixed events and milestones (prepare agenda for meeting by 10th month, ward sisters submit budget items by September 30th, staff appraisal meeting with nurses May lst etc.) and from this a more detailed weekly plan. At the end of each shift a list of tasks emerging from the shift together with tasks indicated by the weekly plan can be made. The list will probably contain too much to accomplish during the next shift, therefore a priority rating will have to be given to each.

AAA Related to key results area. Not possible to delegate to others, must be done immediately
AA   Related to key results — might delegate or could be deferred for a day more
A   Not related to key results — could be delegated or not pressing.

Then the AAA tasks can be roughly allocated to sections of the shift around the normal routines such as ward visits, handover meetings and pre-arranged appointments.

Such a planning system is illustrated on pages 79–81. It would be useful to have a section of your diary or planning dossier with notes on 'bring forward' items (i.e. file memos in sections a week or month ahead when action is required, rather than leave them to pile up in an 'in tray')

It is also time saving to have a data base in this dossier with lists of telephone numbers, addresses and useful references, to reduce the time spent in hunting out such information from various other files.

Managing interruptions

It is not possible to be a good time manager without regular reviews of work problems and effectiveness with colleagues, staff and immediate seniors. By increasing awareness of each other's priorities, mutual planning and delegation, all members of a unit team can be careful in the use of their own time and sensitive to the dangers of wasting other people's time.

The various strategies that are usually recommended in trying to cope with the hazard of interruptions in work, therefore, are only effective if others understand what you are doing and why you are doing it. Given this basic requirement, the list of suggestions below should be of practical application by nurse managers, but more particularly by those in more senior posts.

— Plan each day to include a 'non-available period'.
— Reduce visibility/availability by having a private area or hideaway.
— Reduce amount of time spent walking about.
— Ask for more advance notice of meetings etc.
— Whenever interrupted by caller/telephone check the reason and assess the importance to yourself and the 'interrupter'. Suggest another appointment if lower priority than current work task.
— Be less helpful to others.
— Be less nosey about work of others/events.

Self-discipline and desk management

With proper attention to work planning, a manager is able to exercise control over the events of each working day. The intention then is to apply concentrated efforts to raise personal productivity to an optimum level.

There are a number of general guidelines indicating good working habits which, although only common sense, could be useful to nurse managers trying to cope with heavy workloads.

— Never postpone important matters because they are unpleasant.
— Establish a routine, scheduling definite times for routine matters.
— Do jobs requiring mental effort when you are at your best.
— Fix deadlines for all jobs and stick to them.
— Put off everything that is not important.
— On odd occasions analyse your interruptions and take steps to avoid them or diminish their effect.
— Do one thing at a time.
— Plan your telephone calls whenever possible.
— Use definite times and meetings for discussing routine matters with colleagues.
— Be selective. Learn to say no.
— Make it a regular rule to check your use of time to see if you could have used it better and how.
— Avoid taking work home unless you are certain you will do it.
— Establish realistic work goals.
— Throw away anything you know you will do nothing about.
— Go through your drawers at regular intervals.
— When you are interrupted put the papers you are working on back in the drawer where they belong before approaching a fresh task.
— Do the tasks requiring less mental effort when you are not in the mood for thinking or when you have got only ten minutes, or when there is a high risk of interruption.
— File each piece of paper immediately in the right place.
— Only have one thing at a time on your desk. The task of the moment.
— Systematic approach to 'in tray' — scan all items by speed reading.
— Use priorities: A Immediate attention; B Next attention; C File; D Discard.

Delegating effectively

In theory every individual, from the most senior general manager to the lowest paid employee in an organisation, has specific responsibilities and tasks which make up her particular job and has appropriate authority to use resources and make decisions to achieve the results expected. In this way, a diminishing amount of authority and responsibility are delegated down an organisation.

In practice, organisations do not operate as mechanically and precisely. It is not possible or desirable to define exactly what each job holder needs to do. There is a continuous need for improvement as well as changes in demand which create alterations in job aims and activities. Individuals have different levels of ability and commitment so that some are able and willing to take heavier work-loads than others.

Thus, managing at any level in any organisation incorporates delegating — that is passing to others, responsibility and authority to undertake agreed pieces of work — rather than simply leaving others to fill their jobs as best they can whilst you get on with yours.

It is possible to identify two main purposes for delegation. One can be termed 'operational', where the aims are to get the work-load of a section completed as efficiently as possible. The other is 'development', where the intention is to help particular individuals improve their knowledge, skills and outlook by deliberately giving tasks of greater responsibility. Ideally, managers should try to combine the two aims simultaneously.

There is the need to encourage some nurses to fill their proper role as fully as possible so that responsibility is fairly distributed. Some nurses have a greater propensity to ask for instructions and advice, even in matters which could rightfully be regarded as within their own competence. Some staff need more direction than others, being more liable to error or lacking initiative. Here a ward sister needs to adopt 'a coaching' manner (see Ch. 19) when dealing with such staff. When asked for instruction, instead of explaining or instructing she should ask the staff members for their view of the correct solution and confirm that their answer is correct, or offer guidance if it is not. Then the ward sister should give positive encouragement to the nurses only to refer similar problems in future if they are concerned about the outcome. Thus delegation is not only giving others work tasks, but is also progressively helping others to fulfil their current duties with greatest autonomy and skill. Staff with potential should be given the chance to 'act up' in the next more senior role, either by taking on specific parts or standing in for the job holder for a limited period.

Delegation seems to be such self-evident common sense that it is surprising that any managers could be regarded as poor delegators. Yet one of the most common complaints about managers is weakness in this respect.

The reasons are worth examination. Many managers are inflicted with a reluctance to delegate, only passing tasks to others in a haphazard manner.

Reluctance to delegate can be caused when a senior nurse has been promoted but remains too involved with the activities of her original role. Although this is an understandable tendency in wanting to do things that you are good at rather than pass them to others who might be less competent, it is a danger that all managers need to review carefully. It can be argued that you should delegate such work tasks to others as these are the ones you find easiest to explain and to monitor.

Reluctance to delegate can be an expression of fear. Some managers express the need to be in direct control of their unit by doing as much as possible themselves. Other managers have little confidence in subordinates, take on a heavy personal work-load, and so set up a self-perpetuating cycle.

Under pressure there is a temptation to do something yourself as it is quicker than briefing others.

Thus a desire to be an all-singing all-dancing nurse manager with a low regard for the abilities and motivation of others will lead a manager to be an ineffectual delegator.

If a manager is properly disposed towards the advantages of delegation then it is simple to develop the art of the delegator. The main aim is to reach mutual agreement with someone else on the best way to share the responsibilities and activities for completing some work tasks.

The questions 'Should I do this work?' 'Should others do it?' 'Can others do this work?' are the starting point. If the answer is that others 'should', then the task is to ensure that they 'can'. In an open approach a manager should follow nine simple steps:

1. Reach agreement with someone else on the mutual benefit of them taking on the work task.
2. Ensure that a recognisable chunk of work is to be delegated.
3. Give adequate briefing on the aims and targets for the work.
4. Encourage the other person to work out the method of achieving the aims and feasible deadlines.
5. Check on the validity of chosen method if needed.
6. Agree means of monitoring — control by exception or agreed milestones for reporting.
7. Provide adequate resources and authority for the tasks.
8. Review progress according to agreed terms of monitoring.
9. Debrief on completion of tasks to reinforce learning experience.

This approach makes delegation an open and positive act. This avoids the common errors of senior staff of dumping work on others without adequate briefing or monitoring of resources, or just giving someone little tasks to do like a personal assistant, rather than a complete area of work.

Giving clear instructions

There are circumstances when it is necessary for a manager to direct a member of staff to carry out a particular task where the individual requires precise instruction. Thus being able to give clear directives is an important component of delegation and the effective use of time.

The first requirement in achieving clarity in instructing others is to be clear yourself by some simple planning and preparation.

There is a check list of questions which can be used in such planning:

— What needs to be done?
— Why does it need to be done?
— What should the end result be?
— How could it be done?
— When should it be done?
— When should it be completed?
— Who should be involved?
— Who should be responsible?
— What communication problems are there? (Problems of ability and attitude of staff and language problems, location, shift working etc.)
— Where should the instructions be given?
— What is the best way of giving instruction? (Verbal, verbal and written, written only, face to face, telephone)

Assuming an appropriate identification of the need and purpose of the instructions and the staff to carry them out has been achieved, the planning of the communication aspect should start by considering who the staff are, what they are like and any potential communication barriers.

If the decision is to provide instruction by verbal means, either face to face or by telephone, it is also necessary to follow a systematic routine which will overcome potential problems of receiving and understanding. One simple pattern to follow has six basic stages:

1. Warn receiver that a message is about to be delivered, rather than launch straight into the topic.
2. Give notice of topic. To gain further attention explain what the message is about before going into it. 'It's about Mrs Jones in Bed 3 and the treatment she's been having.'
3. Present the message. Now give the instructions on action that needs to be carried out. Here it may be important to explain the reasons if this improves acceptance and develops knowledge. It will be necessary to state the end result expected, when it should be done, any reporting back required and possibly how it is to be done.
4. Check understanding. Feedback is required to ensure that the receiver understands the why, what, when and any how that has been given.
5. Check action. Further feedback is required to ensure that the receiver has the skill, time and resources necessary to achieve the result and whether any further instruction on the 'how' is needed.
6. Reinforce the key points. To reduce the possibility of errors even further there should be a concluding summary of the main points of instruction.

This may seem rather an elaborate process for simple messages, but for many managers it is a natural routine which will ensure that misunderstandings are eliminated. The feedback (or check) phase can be made more or less elaborate depending on the complexity of the message and the reliability of the receiver. Asking the direct closed questions 'Do you understand?' and 'Can you manage that?' do not give the opportunity for the receiver to ask questions or explain problems, and straight answers 'Yes' do not necessarily give a manager complete reassurance.

Where there is doubt it will be necessary to obtain more feedback by asking detailed and open questions (see Ch. 8), either to get the receiver to repeat the key points or outline how it will be carried through in practice.

The reinforce stage can also be more or less elaborate, ranging from a simple verbal summary to a full repeat with written notes and an indication of the control process (report back, inspection visit etc.) to be employed.

These five basic stages can and should be used when passing on an instruction. The main problem is usually in feedback and reinforcement, and these account for most breakdowns. A ward sister is too busy to check that instructions have been understood; a nurse manager discourages discussion of contentious issues from fear of losing control; a director of nursing telephones several ward sisters but has no mechanism of checking clearly that they have all understood the message. In such circumstances the manager

DAY	Subject/Job						
1							
2							
3							
4							
5							
6							
7							
8							
9							
10							
11							
12							
13							
14							
15							
16							
17							
18							
19							
20							
21							
22							
23							
24							
25							
26							
27							
28							
29							
30							
31							

Fig. 7.1 Monthly plan.

cannot be certain that understanding and action will be the outcome of her attempt at communicating.

We have implied that delegation is only appropriate with immediate subordinate staff. In practice we can share work with several others. Where senior staff are passing on work that they 'should' do to juniors who are already overloaded, the junior might need to pass the work back by 'upward delegation', or when work could be done by colleagues in other sections, 'sideways delegation' can be appropriate.

An effective delegator checks each major

	Month: Week no:
DAY	Week from: to: Activities
MO	
TU	
WE	
TH	
FR	
SA	
SU	

Fig. 7.2 Weekly plan.

work activity by asking 'Should I be doing this all myself?' 'Should/Could others do all or part of it?' 'Would they benefit from this?' 'Should/Could this be delegated?'

When positive answers emerge, delegation is clearly appropriate. This gives a nurse

manager an opportunity of getting a balance in work activities: she can spend some time on high level work appropriate to the seniority of her post, but balance this work with some time spent working alongside subordinate staff as a deliberate act of support

Times	Day plan: tasks for today in order	Day	Tasks carried over	Date
			Tasks from week/month plan	

Fig. 7.3 Day plan: Enter fixed appointments from diary with start/finish times. Enter times for daily routine tasks. Enter times for tasks carried over from previous day. Enter tasks from weekly/monthly plans.

showing solidarity and interest, rather than as an act of exception or as an expedient means of overcoming failures in planning.

IMPROVING TIME MANAGEMENT IN PRACTICE

We have given detailed attention to the problems of planning and controlling use of time in work as it is an essential requirement for anyone who wishes to achieve results in a job and to reduce stress, as well as wishing to achieve more from a career and from life generally.

If you are already in a post with time pressures, it may seem that some of the points we have discussed are relevant, but difficult to see how they can be applied. Improving time management, like improving managerial effectiveness in general, is an act of self-development in which a manager needs to diagnose personal effectiveness and identify tangible means of improving in weak areas.

The start of this process can be self-appraisal in the four main aspects of time management — planning, delegating, self-discipline and coping with interruptions. Select one where improvement is desired and make positive plans to effect the improvement. An alternative start can be to keep a log of how time is spent at present, and to analyse this data to suggest ways of eliminating major time-wasting practices.

Time planning systems

To plan each day effectively it is necessary to include tasks from key results areas and long-term activities with those emerging from on-going work activities and daily routines. It is useful to make an outline monthly and weekly plan with some predictable activities and commitments emerging from longer-term goals and projects. A daily plan will incorporate these as appropriate, together with tasks carried over from the previous day and, ideally, some uncommitted time for unexpected events. Planning forms used alongside a normal diary will form a simple time planning system (see Fig. 7.1; 7.2; 7.3).

REFERENCES

Ferner J 1980 Successful time management. John Wiley & Sons, Chichester
Garratt S 1985 Managing your time. Fontana/Collins, London
Pedler M, Boydell T 1985 Managing yourself. Fontana/Collins, London

Business need for communication

Corporate communication

The barriers
  Size and structure
  Dispersal
  Management attitudes

Communication media

8
Management communication

All organisations are designed essentially as networks for communication amongst the people employed and with those outside who have an interest in the purpose and activities of the organisation. It is part of the responsibilities of all managers to ensure that the necessary communication with seniors, with supervisors, with staff as well as with such outside groups as clients, suppliers, supporters, trade unions and government departments, is carried out successfully.

Communication can be defined as the act of exchanging information (facts, ideas, feelings) with other people so that understanding is achieved. The type of information and the level of understanding required in an organisation is extremely wide but can be summarised in two basic categories which can be distinguished as 'business need' and 'corporate need'.

BUSINESS NEED FOR COMMUNICATION

There is an essential need for information that is accurate and is available at the right time so that all members of an organisation can carry out the tasks of their jobs efficiently. This basic 'business' information can be provided in a variety of verbal, written and pictorial forms. In a hospital this would include all information needed: to ensure that patients are admitted, treated and discharged efficiently; to ensure that all staff know when, where, what and how they are expected to work each day or night; to ensure that all necessary resources are provided and maintained internally (medicines, equipment, food, bedding, etc.) for patient care and staff requirements; to ensure that all goods and services to be supplied to the hospital are delivered in the right quantity, quality and time required; to ensure that all the financial obligations of the health authority are discharged properly (staff payment, suppliers' invoices processed, monies obtained from DHSS, etc.). Clearly in a large hospital, just to provide such essential information will require a highly planned system together with a considerable amount of administrative time and effort producing hundreds of items of information such as:

— Patient admission notes
— Patient records
— Patient appointment notices
— Treatment records
— Routine work instruction
— Operating theatre lists
— Staff rotas
— Temporary staff requisitions
— Stores requisitions
— Budget summaries
— Cost statements
— Job descriptions
— Contracts of employment
— Codes of conduct etc.

Many of these items of information are intended for internal circulation. Some are also directed externally to patients, relatives, doctors, social services, volunteers, etc. All have specific and limited purposes which together are essential if a hospital is to fulfil its purpose.

CORPORATE COMMUNICATION

Even more information is needed, however, if a hospital is to be fully efficient in caring for patients, as well as being a satisfactory place in which to work and to fulfil its overall

community role. Thus, in common with business and public service organisations a health care organisation will need a considerable amount of more general 'corporate' communication. This includes general information dispensed to all staff so that they can better understand health authority policies, procedures, developments and plans; information to assist with staff induction, staff training, professional education and professional updating. Much of this corporate 'propaganda' is essentially one-way communication (from the top management downwards) and is intended to help develop not only an understanding of the health care system in which staff work but also to encourage them to feel more committed towards it. If corporate communication consists of solely one-way traffic, however, and is clearly perceived as propaganda, it is unlikely to achieve this purpose.

There is an essential need to consult with and actively involve staff and managers so that information, suggestions, proposals, grievances and disputes are communicated directly, or via representatives, to the most senior levels of hospital and health authority management.

Corporate communication should also have an outward looking element. There is a public relations need to inform the community about services, developments and plans. As a public service there is also a requirement to consult with representatives of community interest groups. In the independent sector there is a need to 'sell' services to doctors and potential patients.

Some of the most common complaints voiced by staff and middle managers in health care and most other organisations are about gaps and failures in management communication.. Thus the key task of senior hospital managers in common with senior executives running large businesses should be to review the effectiveness of their 'business' and 'corporate' communication. This should result in policies emphasising the need for good communication and planned means for achieving this in practice.

Management communication / 85

THE BARRIERS

Some organisations have more effective communication than others. This may be because there are fewer fundamental problems to be overcome but it can also be a result of greater attention and skill being employed by management. The most common barriers which inhibit the flow of reliable and useful information inside an organisation can be summarised as:

Size and structure
Dispersal
Management attitudes and culture.

Size and structure

It is obviously more difficult for the general manager of a regional health authority to communicate with all nursing staff in the region than it is for a director of nursing services in one hospital. The larger the organisation the greater the likelihood of gaps and failures in communication, although this is not an inevitable consequence of size.

The potential communication problems can be overcome by a management hierarchy that is structured in an appropriate way. If the regional general manager has an appropriate span of control, if each manager through the nursing functions also has appropriate spans of control and there are an appropriate number of layers of managers and supervisors between region and ward level, the problems of size can be overcome.

Dispersal

A communication problem that is often associated with larger organisations is that of having a work-force dispersed over a large area. District health authorities have staff working in different hospitals and many hospitals often have units spread over a wide area. There will also be nursing staff who spend most of their time working in the community. This physical distance will present a barrier to easy and regular information

exchange which has to be overcome by health care and nursing managers. Other practical difficulties which need to be managed are those presented by shift and night working, and the existence of specialist units or departments which are rather outside the main organisation.

Management attitudes

In some work places these practical problems are compounded by an apparent premium on secrecy. Staff have to ask for information; supervisors are only given minimum information. The culture seems to be one where withholding information is the norm rather than disclosure and the development of an 'open' system. This tone is set by senior managers believing that non-disclosure is the most expedient policy, possibly because they are unsure of their authority or from a fear that information might be used against them by trade unions, suppliers, competitors, political or community pressure groups. Some senior managers are simply unaware of the benefits of an open approach to communication.

Middle and junior managers can also be a substantial communication block. They may be informed and involved by more senior managers in planning and development discussions but they do not continue the process with junior staff, either from a need to boost their ego or because of lethargy.

Organisations where individuals feel insecure are likely to be places where secrecy prevails and where people rely on rumours to fill the gap in information. Insecurity will block the flow of communication from the lower levels to the top and from one section to another. This will result in poor decision-making and poor collaboration.

Thus the onus is on senior health care management, both in general management and in senior nurse roles, to develop a management philosophy based on a belief in the virtues of 'open' systems, then to appreciate the practical problems that will inhibit the development of such a system, select the appropriate media to overcome them and ensure that this media is used skilfully.

COMMUNICATION MEDIA

Management has a choice in the means by which information can be delivered and exchanged. These can be grouped into five main categories:

1. Face to face
2. Written
3. Consultative
4. Audio-visual
5. Technological.

Nurse managers need to be conversant with the uses and problems of these different media and to develop personal skills in their selection and use.

In considering the topic of management communication we have started with a broad account of the range of media at the disposal of senior management to create a comprehensive communications system. Although it is clear that the responsibility for developing and maintaining such a system rests with general managers at regional, district and unit level, specialised nurse managers also have important communication responsibilities.

REFERENCES

Porritt L 1984 Communication choices for nurses. Churchill Livingstone, Edinburgh
Savendra M, Hawthorne J 1984 Supervision. Pan, London

Personal communication network

Personal communication skills
  Lack of interest — lack of attention
  Retention — shared language
  Assumptions
  Prejudices
  Lack of trust
  Use of intermediaries
  Time

9

Nurse managers as communicators

Senior nurses should be aware of the communication system in their organisations and know of the sources of information that are relevant to their own activities. Where they identify aspects of communication policy or practice that are inadequate they should make reasoned proposals for improvement. At the same time they must ensure that they are personally competent as communicators.

In this respect nurse managers have to be more than just conveyors of information. They are team leaders, trainers of staff, advisors to colleagues, members of a management team, members of a health care team, advisors to doctors, counsellors to patients and their relatives and members of the nursing profession. This multifarious role requires communication skill in the complete sense — being able to understand others, getting them to understand you, relating to others as human beings as well as employees of a large bureaucracy. Communication is the essential ingredient for effective team work and satisfactory human relationships.

It is useful for an individual manager to consider the extent of her current communications network, to assess whether it is extensive enough, or too extensive, and whether the quality of information exchange needs to be improved.

87

PERSONAL COMMUNICATION NETWORK

The term 'network' refers to all the personal contacts that have to be made in the process of obtaining and giving information. Some of these contacts are with subordinate staff in a manager's formal 'area of responsibility'. Other, just as vital contacts are with services and colleagues where influence is necessary but where authority is either non-existent or ambiguous. These may be regarded as being in the 'area of influence'. A third element of a network will be those contacts which can be used as 'sources of information'. The important issue, however, is for senior nurses to acknowledge that they have to influence other people over whom they have little direct authority, and have to build up informal contacts for advice and to keep them informed when the official communication systems are likely to be inadequate.

The basis for being fully competent and influential in any professional or managerial job, is having an appropriate communication network and a system for using the network effectively.

In the section on organising your own work and managing time (Ch. 7) we suggest a practical method of planning. Thus a simple plan by a senior nurse for communicating will involve appropriate time for the obvious activities of ward visits, staff meetings, individual coaching sessions, teaching, visits to senior nurses, as well as for fixed commitments like unit meetings, doctors' rounds and for the less regular contacts with community groups, trade union representatives, personnel officers, senior tutors, etc. By systematic planning a proper balance might be achieved within the individual's network rather than simply responding to current demands of others.

Part of the process of planning would involve selecting the best media for communication. This means answering such questions as: 'Is it better to have daily meetings in the office with senior ward staff or make ward rounds twice a shift?' 'Is it better to have duplicated copies of important instructions handed to all members of staff or just display one copy on a notice board?' 'Should minutes of unit meetings be circulated?' 'Is the ward procedures manual accessible and understood?'

This planned system then requires a nurse manager/communicator to use personal skill to turn every contact into a fruitful encounter, or to use media in a way that will transfer information appropriately.

PERSONAL COMMUNICATION SKILLS

We have described an organisation with free-flowing information as an 'open' system. At the level of communication between individuals and small groups there is a similar need for openness if mutual understanding is to be achieved and unambiguous messages are to be transmitted and received. Openness between ward sister and senior nurse, between ward sister and nurses means that individuals genuinely try to understand each other. Unfortunately there are many barriers which can close down interpersonal communication and cloud understanding.

All acts of communication have 'presenters' and 'receivers' of information (messages). In two-way communication (conversations, exchange of correspondence) the role of presenter/receiver switches between individuals. There are a number of common barriers which hinder satisfactory transfer:

1. Lack of interest in content of message by one or both parties
2. Lack of attention during communication, mind wandering in meetings, notices not fully read, etc.
3. Lack of retention by receivers who listen to message but forget parts later
4. Lack of shared language between parties; jargon or technical language not understood
5. Wrong assumptions by either party, assuming existing knowledge, attitudes, etc.
6. Prejudices and predisposition by either party, thus not being prepared to listen to others' opinions

Exercise 1

Nurse Manager Network   Self Assessment

1. List in the space below the individuals and groups with whom you make contact now.
2. Consider whether the quality of your communication with any individuals or groups needs to be improved, i.e. more time, more contact, better understanding.
3. Consider whether this list needs to be extended to improve your effectiveness.

Area of responsibility

Present contact	Effectiveness				Possible improvement
	Excellent	Generally good	Needs improvement	Very poor	

Possible extensions
(Who should you add to your network in the area of responsibility)

Area of influence

Present contacts | Effectiveness | Possible improvement

Excellent | Generally good | Needs improvement | Very poor

Possible extensions
(Who should you add to your network in the area of influence)

Sources of information

Present contacts		Effectiveness		Possible improvement
Excellent	Generally good	Needs improvement	Very poor	

Possible extensions
(Who should you add to your network in the area of influence

7. Lack of trust by receiver, thus discrediting the message content; conflicts of interest between parties, preventing open-minded consultation of each others' message
8. Using intermediaries, leading to distortion of messages passed from one to another
9. Authority differences between parties inhibiting the free exchange of information
10. Inappropriate time/timing so that receiver is unwilling to consider message.

Lack of interest — lack of attention

Before information can be passed successfully from one person to another the 'receiver' must be prepared, or be persuaded, to give sufficient attention to the message so that it can be understood. Therefore, when writing a report, preparing a training session or informally explaining the operation of a new procedure, try to express the content in a way that will grab the interest and attention of the receivers. Although this is obvious, many managers either assume wrongly that others share their fascination with a particular topic or only express themselves in extremely dull fashion.

Such problems not only threaten the effectiveness of basic one-way communication, but also have a bearing on what are intended as more participative meetings. A manager wrongly assumes that ward staff will be excited by the prospect of listening to an analysis of budgets and costs and will then join in a fruitful two-way debate. However, unless such information is well presented and some thought given to a means of stimulating discussion this is unlikely to happen.

Retention — shared language

Words are the building blocks of communication, but for understanding to be achieved people have to share a similar way of using the same words. At the simplest level, many health care organisations employ a multi-racial work-force where many individuals will be using English as a second language. Even between native English speakers there will be different levels of comprehension and differences of interpretation. Business, technical and professional communication is peppered with jargon and specialised vocabulary. We do not always understand each others' jargon or share the same technical vocabulary (software, ECG, off-duty rota, hands-on experience, nursing process, behaviour modification, region, etc.).

Words also have emotional content which lead to different interpretations. 'Profit', 'value for money', 'cost effective' have a desirable connotation to some but not to others; similarly such words as 'new technology', 'rationalisation', 'redeployment', 'administration' have very different meanings for different individuals.

Thus managers seeking to communicate with each other across different sections in the same organisation, as well as communicating with staff or trade union representatives, will have to assess the extent to which the language they use will be understood.

Obviously some people find learning and remembering easier than others. This is partly due to differences in ability and differences in interest in particular subject matter. At the end of a meeting or training session it is certain that nobody can recall 100% of information exchanged. As time elapses the amount retained will reduce rapidly.

The retention problem is not just about difficulty in remembering, however, but also about interpretation. Each witness at an accident has a different impression of what happened. Participants at a meeting will bring their own set of interests and values to bear so that they remember selectively, and will often distort what was said by others so that it fits into their own frame of reference more comfortably.

Assumptions

Unambiguous instructions are extremely difficult to write. Presenting a training session in which learners are able to grasp fully the content is also difficult. One of the main problems is that the communicator has to make assumptions about the general ability level and existing knowledge of the receivers. If these are underestimated the messages are full of unnecessary explanation and instruction; if these are overestimated the receiver will soon find himself lost.

Ideally, a manager should be aware of the ability, knowledge and skills of others she wishes to instruct or to persuade, so that the content, style, manner and vocabulary can be selected accordingly.

Prejudices

We all have strongly held opinions on many issues. Some beliefs can be so strong that they blind us to the possibility that they may be incorrect. Such convictions, considered from other people's perspectives, become prejudices and biases which close our mind to different points of view or new situations. Where individuals meet to discuss issues in work about which there are already strong feelings it is likely that discussion degenerates into argument, deadlock and confrontation.

In many hospitals there are differences in view between some consultants and some senior nurses on the appropriate role of nurses. There may be different views between catering officers and ward sisters on the most effective ways to feed patients. Shop stewards will view the introduction of privatisation of services differently from hospital administrators.

This does not mean that health service staff are more difficult or prejudiced than other people. All organisations have groups and individuals with strongly opposing outlooks as well as issues on which most agree. This fact of organisational life means that nurse managers will need to consider the effect that others' prejudices will have on any topics about which they wish to communicate.

If managers wish others to treat them in a constructive and open-minded way they must be prepared to be constructive and open-minded themselves. If you are trying to sell new ideas you must be prepared to have others question the validity of your ideas and

be prepared to understand the reasons for their objections. This requires a tolerant and patient approach to others.

Lack of trust

Managers often complain that staff are unwilling to inform them when things go wrong. They prefer to cover up rather than admit faults. Bad news is often withheld from senior managers. There is a natural tendency for most of us to wish to be seen in a favourable light by seniors, colleagues and staff. Without deliberately lying it is likely that we will present interpretations of facts and events which confirm our good image.

In most organisations, minor distortions and censorship will be inevitable barriers to open communication which managers must learn to cope with. In some organisations distortion becomes more extreme leading to a serious lack of trust between various individuals and groups. The transmission of messages and development of mutual understanding is not possible without trust. If staff have learned that some managers do not keep their word, or say one thing while doing another, this will seriously disrupt further communication and working relationships.

Use of intermediaries

It can be easily demonstrated that the more times a message is passed from one individual to another the more distortion and inaccuracy there is. If the practice in a hospital is for information to be relayed from a unit management meeting to senior nurses' meeting and then to individual ward sisters and finally to ward staff, there will be several intermediaries in the chain.

Even if each link in this communication is well-intentioned, it is certain that some ward sisters would get different messages and some would probably receive nothing at all. It is likely that several of the intermediaries will be under pressure, will have strong views about the issues and will have staff on different shifts and other practical problems, thus making distortion and loss of content even more of a serious matter.

Time

We all experience the problem of trying to talk to someone who is distracted and unable to give us full attention. Often this is simply because we have chosen the wrong moment to raise a particular issue. Thus choosing the right time for meetings is a significant consideration. Some managers deliberately call staff meetings towards the end of a shift, or just before a meal break, as they know this will tend to restrict discussion. Others have meetings early in the day so that there will be no artificial time restraint. We need to choose the right time to talk to individual staff or senior colleagues so that the 'moment' is appropriate and amount of time is consistent with the nature of our business.

From an examination of these potential barriers it is possible to suggest some general communication guidelines for nurse managers. It is useful to distinguish between the acts of interpersonal, face-to-face communication and those relying more on the written word.

Interpersonal communication: the key points
- Pay attention
- Avoid side-tracking
- Be patient
- Use silence
- Make notes

10
Effective interpersonal communication

The most common form of communicating for line managers in nursing will be face to face, involving a wide variety of encounters with individuals and small groups.

As we all spend such a large portion of our lives talking with other people it should not be necessary to advise managers and supervisors on the approaches to effective questioning and listening. This is especially pertinent for trained staff in the health care profession whose basic craft depends on an ability to understand other people and to be understood by them. Yet all nursing staff will have personal experience of working with managers who seem unwilling to listen, preferring to talk at others instead of engaging in constructive two-way discussion.

At the start of any conversation in work and throughout its duration a manager needs to be sensitive to others involved. Sensitivity means being aware of the feelings of others, thinking about their motivations, understanding the impact we have on others and how their behaviour in turn affects us, rather than simply thinking of our own problems and being determined to put across 'our' message irrespective of the opinions and wishes of others.

Thus a senior nurse who starts a conversation with a ward sister: 'I know that you have been under pressure this week and I'm very grateful for how you have coped. I am certain that you'll get two students next week, but I'm afraid that we'll be short-staffed again until then,' is showing some consideration of her problem which is not evident if she started the conversation in an alternative manner: 'The acute unit is short-staffed again, so I'm under pressure as usual, and I'll have to pinch Nurse Jones from you . . .'

Of course the only really sensitive start is to invite the ward sister to talk about the circumstances in her ward first. This will give an understanding of any problems she has and an appreciation of her current feelings which can be taken into account in the subsequent discussion.

Such sensitivity will be displayed further by good questioning and listening skills. In theory a question is a request by one person for information from another. For this aim to be achieved, in practice, it is helpful to phrase the request in a way that encourages the other person to respond appropriately. There is a basic choice between asking 'closed' and 'open' questions. A closed question is worded in a way that suggests that only a one word answer is required. An open question is worded in a way that suggests a more expansive reply is appropriate.

Thus in the conversation described earlier, the senior nurse should end her statement with a question so that she obtains feedback from the ward sister. Some closed questions would be:

'Is that alright?'
'Do you understand my problem?'
'Will that give you enough cover?'
'You'll cope with that, will you?'

Alternatively, more open questions would be:

'How do you feel about that?'
'What problems does that cause you?'
'How much cover will that give you?'
'How will you cope with the situation?'

If you want someone else to 'open up', then it is preferable to ask open-ended questions. Closed questions should be used when seeking straight answers to unambiguous questions, to check simple facts or as a preliminary to asking further questions.

Thus a conversation will proceed from closed to open questions:

'Is that alright?'
'Not really.'
'What's the problem then?'

When the issues and differences have been aired ideally the senior will have been persuaded to change her plan, or has been able to reassure the ward sister, or there has been mutual agreement on a compromise. As a last resort she may have to instruct the sister and use her authority to impose a decision.

In any event, a conversation will conclude with a closed question which is answered in a way indicating communication has been successful:

'Is that clear?'   ('Yes, it is now.')
'Any other   ('No, I can cope')
problems?'
'Is that acceptable?' ('Yes, I'll do my best.')

Of course in open relationships between people, the choice of question style is of less importance. The question may be closed 'Does that give you enough cover?', but the answer may be open 'No, I'm afraid not, the problem is that we have to provide. . . . .'

It is preferable to use open and closed questions in an appropriate way, but our underlying intentions are of greatest significance. If you are trying to be open-minded and encourage another person to explain his point of view, it is useful to begin questions with: 'what; why; when; where; how; which; who.'

If a manager does not have an open mind, this will be displayed in the way that she uses questions: not really requests for information but attempts to persuade, intimidate or manipulate other people. These managers use 'loaded' or 'leading' questions. These are usually closed and include a suggestion of the answer that is required.

'I know you'll be able to cope with this, is that right?'
'As a responsible person you will accept this?'

'You don't want to cause me any more problems do you?'

'I take it that you can manage your staff OK?'

If you are sensitive to the processes of conversation and aware of your own motives you will notice that you ask closed questions or loaded questions when you really wish to be more 'open' or 'neutral'. This dilemma often arises through lack of self-confidence, pressure of time, uncertainty about prying into other people's feelings, or inexperience in dealing with issues.

This difficulty can be overcome by trying to recover the situation by tagging on a more appropriate conclusion to the question: 'I know you'll be able to cope with this, is that right?' or 'Do you have any difficulties? Please be honest.'

The most likely way of progressing a conversation from such a potential stopping point, however, is by listening carefully to replies and watching 'non-verbal signals'. 'Active' listening means concentrating not only on what the other person is saying, but also on what he is leaving out; what assumptions he is making and what hints he is giving about his feelings and opinions. This means that a conversation progresses by one person asking follow-up questions of the other to get more detailed information, to probe the meaning of what has been said, to encourage him to carry on with his theme or to check that he has finished. Thus the ward sister replies to the question 'Do you have any difficulties?' by saying 'Well, I'm under pressure from Nurse Jones. . .you know she's got this problem at home.'

If the senior nurse is listening she can encourage the sister to explain the circumstances. She can probe by requesting further information:

'What problem does that create for you?' or 'Tell me about Nurse Jones.'

This involves further listening and further probing questions or encouragement to continue. The final evidence that understanding is being achieved is the ability of the listener to feed back in summary his interpretation of the essence of what the other person has expressed. The frustration of trying to talk to someone who fails to grasp your meaning, misinterprets or distorts it is well known. Thus in giving some feedback to check that you have understood someone else in the way *he* has tried to explain his ideas, circumstances, problem or feelings, he will know if some misunderstanding has arisen. He can then try to correct the false impression. Further summary and feedback may then confirm that understanding has been achieved.

It also enables you to play for time. If you are not sure how to answer a question or criticism, or feel that there is potential conflict with the other person try to go back over the main points of his argument. This will help you to think and to avoid unnecessary confrontation.

Concentrating on another person as he is talking or as he is listening, also involves observing his physical actions. Certain body postures suggest certain feelings. If the ward sister is sitting back comfortably looking at the senior nurse whilst nodding and smiling, these are non-verbal signals suggesting agreement. If she is hunched up with clenched hands, shaking her head and has a bleak facial expression, the signals suggest different feelings. Similarly, posture, eye contact, facial expression and tone of voice will add meaning to what someone is saying. There may be consistency between words and gestures (a manager saying that a new project is exciting whilst leaning forward, looking pleased and sounding enthusiastic); or there may be lack of congruence (the same manager using the same phrases but in a dull tone, without animated gestures and a 'laid-back' posture).

Other non-verbal aspects, where participants in conversation place themselves in relation to each other, are standing close and touching, which can be signs of sympathy and encouragement; keeping one's distance, maintaining a desk as a barrier, standing whilst others sit can be gestures that establish distance.

INTERPERSONAL COMMUNICATION: THE KEY POINTS

Pay attention

Do not let your eyes or mind get distracted whilst others are talking. There is a danger of thinking up a reply or counter-argument instead of really listening.

Avoid side-tracking

As you listen to some talk, it inevitably sparks off thoughts and ideas which can be at a tangent or not directly relevant to what is being said. It is important to exercise self-discipline by making a mental or actual note whilst still listening, continue the conversation in a logical sequence but then raise those matters at a more appropriate time.

Be patient

Do not interrupt whilst someone is talking, do not over-ride what he is saying or try to finish off his points for him. If you feel an issue has been covered or is being laboured it is still more sensitive to wait for a gap or for the person to conclude before moving on.

Use silence

If you are trying to draw someone out or to really think through an issue by discussion with someone else, it is useful to let a few seconds elapse after he has stopped talking to see if he has really finished and to allow your mind to explore the matter. Instant responses may be distracting or superficial.

Make notes

If someone is describing a problem or presenting detailed information, making brief notes as he talks will assist concentration and save time lost in having to ask for information that has already been given. Noting a word or two to remind you of points you wish to make or where clarification is needed will prevent unhelpful interruptions. At the end of a conversation, if agreement on action has been reached, this should be noted.

These general considerations about effectiveness in interpersonal communication underpin all face-to-face meetings at work. We therefore assume that the general skills will be practised in all encounters, but there are some common face-to-face situations for managers which need to be considered separately:

— Giving instructions (Ch. 7)
— Meetings (Ch. 11)
— Selection (Ch. 18)
— Counselling and grievance interviewing (Ch. 16)
— Disciplinary interviewing (Ch. 17)
— Staff appraisal and coaching (Ch. 20)
— Consultation and negotiation (Ch. 11)

REFERENCES

Ceccio C, Ceccio J 1982 Effective communication for nursing. John Wiley, New York
French P 1984 Social skills for nurses. Croom Helm, London
Smith, V M, Bass T A 1982 Communication for the health care team. Harper and Row, London
Tappen R 1983 Nursing leadership. F A Davis, Philadelphia

11

Managing meetings

Nurse managers and staff tend to hold rather extreme views about meetings. Many have come to regard them as a waste of time and a distraction from doing 'real' work. A minority hold the alternative view that meetings *are* the real work of management.

If being a manager is about organising the work of others through planning, making decisions, co-ordinating and controlling, the act of face-to-face communication is essential to this purpose. It is not possible to run a health care organisation without consultation between management and staff, or without continuous exchanges of information. These meetings are an essential component of all hospitals and health authority communication systems. Despite this undeniable importance of meetings, in practice a large number are a waste of time and source of irritation to those involved.

PURPOSE OF MEETINGS

A meeting can be a very informal and brief contact between two people, or it can be a ritualistic large-scale committee. Participants in either extreme need to be clear and agreed on the reason for getting together.

There are four distinct purposes for calling a meeting:

Information and briefing

These can be called 'command' meetings in which a senior person (in rank or expertise) convenes a meeting to pass on information, instructions or advice to others. These are essentially one-way communication meetings.

Consultation meetings

These are meetings where the purpose is to interchange information, opinions and advice between all participants. The meeting can be between professional colleagues; between team leaders and their work team; between management representatives and staff or trades union representatives; between health authority representatives and 'community' representatives. These should be two-way or round table discussions but not leading to binding decisions.

Decision-making meetings

As running a Health Service whether at district or ward level is a team activity, many management decisions should be taken either through the process of group meetings or individually after consultative meetings. Thus decision-making meetings are an essential feature of management activities. Such meetings can reach decisions in three alternative ways. One is to debate issues, pool ideas, explore differences until a concensus is reached on a decision (i.e. all agree). The second is for similar debate and discussion but for a decision to be made by majority vote. The third way is for the most senior person to listen to the contribution of all participants, to clarify any major differences and then to impose a decision on the meeting.

Negotiation meetings

Where there is a meeting between individuals of similar standing or equal power representing different sections or interest groups (such as a district personnel officer meeting NUPE representatives on plans to change work practices, or a director of nursing services, medical officer, district general manager, hospital administrator meeting to agree allocation of resources), decisions will have to be made by mutual agreement. This will involve some bargaining and some compromise if there are conflicts of aim or interest between participants.

It is possible in practice to run an effective meeting which has several objectives, if this is understood by all and that each item or phase has a clear purpose. Thus a health care team meeting could have some items which are purely briefing, followed by some which are decision-making. A meeting can conclude with a negotiated agreement on an item of dispute but start with a round table consultative discussion.

EFFECTIVE MEETINGS

The main reasons that meetings are ineffective are insufficient preparation by those involved, and inappropriate leadership by the person responsible for running the meeting.

Preparation

Whether it be a hastily convened meeting between a senior nurse and one ward sister or a formal gathering of a health authority committee, a meeting will benefit from preparation before the event by all who are to be involved. The meeting convenor should be clear before the event about:

— The purpose of the meeting
— The format and constitution
— Who should attend
— Whether an agenda should be circulated
— Where the meeting will be held
— The time it will commence
— How long it should last
— What papers should be distributed beforehand
— What papers and information should be available at the meeting

— Whether 'minutes' will be taken and circulated
— The proposed distribution of minutes.

Decisions on the form and constitution of meetings will define the decision-making authority (can we make binding agreements on expenditure, changes in procedures, etc.?) and the topic that comes within that authority (safety in the hospital, patient meals; ward routines, etc.). There will also be an indication of the process for reaching decisions (majority vote, etc.). If the meeting is consultative without a mandate to make collective decisions it is essential for all attending to be aware of this and accept the limitation.

It is possible to have an effective meeting between two people, or between twenty-two. Clearly, the more attending, the more formal the meeting and the less likely there will be involvement by all. The larger the membership the greater the potential for considering all sides of an issue. The more people attending, however, the more likely it is that many will regard it as a waste of time. In planning a meeting it is important to get the best balance between being too small and unrepresentative and too large. It is generally considered that meetings involving more than a dozen people are likely to be unwieldy and less productive than smaller gatherings.

An individual who is required to attend a meeting should be prepared to question the need and value of her presence. It could be more effective to send a deputy or only attend for selected items on the agenda.

All meetings need a general framework so that discussion can progress in a constructive manner. Thus a leader of an informal meeting or the chairperson in a committee needs to prepare an agenda. In rapidly arranged meetings over urgent problems the 'agenda' need not be distributed beforehand. It is enough that a minute or two is given at commencement to clarify the purpose of the meeting, to indicate the topics to be considered and agree a sensible order to cover them — the 'agenda'. This is essential if time is to be used wisely and decisions are to be made systematically.

In formal meetings or regularly held meetings it is advisable to write an agenda after consultation with interested parties and to send this out before the event. This should be used by participants to prepare information and canvas views of others so that the meeting will be properly informed and concise. There is a danger that having 'any other business' on an agenda will allow individuals to spring items on others or unnecessarily extend a meeting. The leader needs to be wary of this practice and to encourage others to use AOB responsibly, if at all.

The time and place that meetings are held can have a significant bearing on their usefulness. Some managers deliberately arrange meetings towards the end of the day or shift so that participants will be precise in order to end on time. There can be an element of manipulation, however, in artificially restricting the time available for a meeting in order to force decisions without adequate debate. Thus balance is needed between having open-ended meetings where discussion may be drawn out to fill the available time, and brief, superficial meetings.

It is useful to provide as much information to participants before a meeting as possible. This enables them to read it, to obtain additional information and form some views about important issues. Again, there can be elements of manipulation where information is only provided during a meeting, as this increases the chances of serious points or the full implication of decisions being overlooked.

All meetings need some written record, either prepared at the time or shortly afterwards. At a minimum this is a brief note on actions agreed, the time-scale and who is to undertake them. Formal meetings usually produce more detailed minutes. A common form of minute contains:

— Date of meeting
— Those in attendance
— Apologies for absence

— Summary of main points discussed under each agenda item and decisions agreed
— Date of next meeting.

The amount of detail contained can range from a full verbatim report to a brief summary. The responsibility for issuing minutes rests with the convenor of a meeting, although the actual note taking and writing might be delegated to a meetings 'secretary'. It is useful for all participants to take notes during a meeting, particularly on points of agreement/ disagreement and decisions for action. This will enable them to check the validity of 'official' minutes and whether decisions have been implemented correctly.

Minutes can also serve to inform those not attending a meeting of what has taken place. In this circumstance it can be useful to produce more interesting and easily read accounts of the significant points rather than publish a turgid account of all that took place.

Meeting skills

A well-planned meeting where everyone arrives prepared to deal with the business in hand in a constructive and efficient way is likely to get off to a satisfactory start. Its satisfactory conclusion depends to a large extent on the skills of the leader.

The leader

There are several alternative models to follow when acting as a meeting leader. At one extreme there is the formal committee chairman who exercises fairly strict control on the meeting (introducing each item, selecting who shall speak, restricting contributions, calling for proposals, putting motions to a vote and insisting that everyone addresses remarks 'through the chair'). At the other extreme is the informal facilitator of group discussion. The choice of style should be determined by the purpose and type of meeting to be conducted. Being too formal and chairman-like can reduce the spontaneity and constructive qualities in a group; being too informal can lead to rambling and indecisive meetings. A significant decision is whether as leader you wish to participate in the content of discussion and exercise direct influence over the outcome, or whether you wish to act as 'facilitator' only, ensuring the group processes are constructively directed but not joining in with personal opinions on the content of agenda items.

As formal chairman of a committee-style meeting the role requires:

— Introducing the meeting and starting on time
— Indicating apologies for absence (or asking the committee secretary to do so)
— Obtaining approval of the meeting on the accuracy of minutes from previous meetings
— Introducing matters arising from the minutes
— Introducing the first agenda items or directing a member to give background to the item
— Opening the matter for discussion by asking for views
— Directing individual members to speak who indicate they wish to do so
— Watching for indications from others
— Possibly restricting each member to one contribution or restricting the time allocated for each item
— Asking for information or opinions from members as appropriate
— Answering points of dispute concerning the constitution or conduct of the meeting
— Seeking decisions, either by asking for a proposal and putting this to a vote, or by making a directive to be accepted by the committee
— Directing particular points to be noted in minutes or to be deleted from the record
— Bringing a meeting to a close and agreeing a date and time of a further meeting.

In very formal committees all contributions are directed 'through the chair' so that individuals do not engage in cross talk. In less formal meetings the chairman will allow such inter-group discussion.

The skills of a chairman are:

— To be able to introduce items so that all members understand the content and purpose
— To stimulate constructive contributions by asking effective questions
— To prevent side-tracking and repetition by members
— To allow enough time and deviation so that items are properly considered
— To summarise key points raised and suggest ways of avoiding deadlock
— To summarise points and actions agreed, and ensure that those responsible will carry out these actions after the meeting.

It is difficult to combine the role of chairman in a large meeting and be an active participant in debating issues and problems. Where the leader adopts this dual role it leads to domination and considerable one-way traffic rather than group discussion and group decision-making.

The role of leader in more informal groups or team meetings is less defined than in committee chairmanship. The main requirements are:

— Introduce the meeting by clarifying the purpose
— Outline an appropriate 'agenda' if one has not been issued
— Seek agreement from the rest on the purpose and suitability of the agenda
— Introduce item one
— Direct appropriate member to give necessary background information
— Invite questions, opinions or suggestions from others
— Prevent domination by more assertive members
— Ask for necessary information and views from all as appropriate
— Allow group interchange if constructive
— Try to encourage open expression of views, concerns and differences
— Seek to resolve conflicts by questioning underlying reasons for differences and suggesting appropriate compromises

— Summarise points and issues and alternatives so that group can progress towards concensus decisions
— Clarify decisions made, actions agreed and who is to be responsible to carry them out
— Make notes of key points or direct someone else to keep this record
— Close the meeting.

The effectiveness of a meeting can be assessed by the extent to which the communication purpose was achieved, if any practical actions were agreed and carried out in practice. If the role of leader is crucial to effectiveness, the responsibility is not his or hers alone.

The participant

In committees there will be a need for a secretary to keep an accurate record of proceedings so that accurate minutes can be produced. In the most formal committees the secretary takes no part in the process or content of the meeting. In less formal meetings it is possible to combine the task of note taking with participation, but it is difficult and this is sometimes used as a device to inhibit an over-assertive individual. In the variety of ad hoc meetings that are essential for the smooth running of any organisation, it is good practice for any actions that have been agreed to be noted briefly by at least one participant. This can be confirmed by a simple memo if the item is of significance or cannot be carried out immediately.

One of the main reasons for managers and staff complaining about meetings is the lack of clarity at the conclusion or outcome and the lack of follow-up to ensure that promises are fulfilled.

Everyone involved in a meeting, however small and casual, has a responsibility to contribute in as informed and concise a way as possible. This reduces time-wasting, and improves communication and decision-making. You should be clear about the purpose of any meeting you attend. If this is not evident from invitations or agendas, or stated by the leader at the outset, then participants should seek clarification before the proceedings get underway. If warning of a meeting has been given then you should give an appropriate time for preparation. Study the agenda, identify information that you need to make a worthwhile contribution, discuss with others who are interested to obtain views and make some notes. If you have items for the agenda, more detailed preparation may be required. Such preparation may only take a few minutes, but will make a significant difference to the conduct of meetings. It also demonstrates to others your effectiveness and will enhance your reputation with staff, colleagues and seniors.

Some individuals find it hard to assert themselves in the often abrasive atmosphere of organisational meetings. If this is your problem, preparation will help as you will be more confident at the start. If you make a determined effort to get in early at a meeting this makes your presence felt and increases self-confidence. It is essential to participate in a meeting when not actually speaking, however. Listen to others, take some notes to ensure you recall the main points, note your thoughts as they occur and the main areas of any disagreement; this will mean that all members keep up with the progress of a meeting. One of the most irritating features of meetings is an individual who shows he has not been listening by asking questions or going over ground already covered. The more introverted individual can be most effective by listening carefully, thinking about a problem whilst others are arguing it out, and coming in quietly with a summary and suggested solution when others have reached an impasse.

When a group is involved in regular meetings it is a worthwhile practice to review the need for the meetings and their effectiveness. The leader is best placed to ask the basic questions occasionally:

'Why are we meeting?'
'Are these meetings really necessary?'
'Do we all need to attend?'
'Do we meet too frequently or too infrequently?'

'Can I be more effective as leader?'
'Can we save time?'
'Can we achieve more in our meetings?'
'Could some members improve their contribution?'
'How can we become more effective?'

In this way managers can apply the principles of effective management (being clear on objectives, getting feedback on performance and identifying means of improvement) to the often wasteful but absolutely essential process of regular face-to-face meetings.

The points we have considered are applicable to all forms of meetings involving nurses and nurse managers. There are some additional special considerations which are relevant to particular types of meetings.

Briefing meetings

The skills to use in running or participating in such meetings are those to be used in giving instructions or making presentations, which have been discussed in Chapters 7 and 18.

Consultation meetings

Exchanging views with other people in work can take the form of senior nurses seeking advice over clinical or managerial problems as well as the gathering of a management team or unit staff for a frank talk about matters of mutual interest or concern. The most contentious form, yet a most important activity, is occasional consultation meetings with staff and trade union representatives.

There can be substantial practical difficulties in setting up meetings with natural work groups, because the work processes, as well as other pressures, usually take priority during normal working hours. It may be possible to hold consultative meetings during lulls, at meal-breaks or at the end of a shift. Alternatively, a series of smaller gatherings can be arranged so that groups of staff are released at a time and 'production' is maintained by the rest.

In many cases, it is not the practical problems that inhibit consultation so much as reluctance on the part of management. This stems from a belief that the task is to control and instruct staff, not to waste time asking for their opinions. It may also be born of experience where employees have not responded to invitations to participate, or have used the opportunity to grouse about management.

Such attitudes can become 'self-fulfilling prophesies' in that a manager who holds a meeting with staff but believes that it is likely to be a waste of time, will conduct the meeting in a way that will ensure it turns out to be a negative experience.

If departmental heads really believe that involving staff is worthwhile as a way of increasing interest, co-operation and better working practices, then they will overcome the practical barriers and derive benefit.

When setting up departmental consultation, management must be prepared for two-way exchanges. They will wish to examine topics of concern to themselves, but should be encouraged to raise issues of interest to their staff as well.

The true spirit of consultation suggests that any topic which concerns participants should be placed on an agenda for discussion. At the local level, however, there will be some constraints on this liberal outlook as there will be limitations in policies or practices. Thus it is important to examine all the potential consultation subjects to identify those appropriate for departmental debate.

Matters of immediate interest to staff as well as their managers may include:

— Working environment (heating, lighting, furniture, layout, etc.)
— Work allocation (job availability, transfers, work-load, etc.)
— Welfare (holidays, social life, sickness, etc.)
— Training and induction
— Equipment and layout
— Nursing standards, methods, quality, plans and development
— Quality control
— Budgets and cost control
— Promotions
— Management authority

— Disciplinary problems
— Work rules and procedures
— Labour turnover and recruitment
— Trade union representation.

The issues that concern local staff are obviously related to wider policies. Some of these will be beyond the scope of departmental influence but can still be of mutual interest:

— Capital investment programmes
— Manpower plans and employment policies
— Operational budgets
— Reorganisation plans
— Take-overs and mergers
— Closures and redundancies
— Purchasing policy, stock levels
— Asset sales
— New technology
— Research and development
— Management appointments and pay.

Such a list will undoubtedly raise doubts and resistance among many managers. There is a traditional reserve in this country about providing information to employees, let alone making time for open debate with them. It may help doubting managers to examine the list of potential consultation topics and allocate each into one of the following categories:

— Can be fully discussed and subject to joint decision without reference to higher authority
— Can be fully discussed but joint decision would need further ratification
— Can be fully discussed but only recommendations for further review or information could be made locally
— Can be discussed in a limited way for information purposes.

It is likely that staff and trade union representatives will have different views on which subjects could be open for full discussion and joint decision-making.

In organisations with a hierarchy of committees, the subject matter for each level can be similar, but the depth of discussion and decision-making authority would diminish at the lower levels.

Genuine consultation requires managers

and staff to be committed to the principle of joint discussion and to have agreed an appropriate formula for carrying out resulting decisions in practice.

Meetings where opinions are openly expressed will reflect the actual state of relations in a particular location. If feelings are critical of management policy and practice, then managers are likely to find meetings rather threatening. They may then act defensively, which makes staff even more destructive. Thus consultative meetings will only improve relations if they actually get to the heart of the causes of existing problems, and if they are conducted in a constructive manner by managers to lead to some practical outcome.

It is particularly important to follow through after a meeting so that agreed actions are completed. Nothing is more likely to create apathy than attending meetings which do not resolve issues.

Consultative committees should be a means of improving understanding between managers and managed, not an end in themselves. There is always the danger that a departmental meeting of selected representatives will act as another elite, rather than a source of wider information. Thus a link back to any staff not directly involved is important.

Given that managers have got the objectives and framework about right, they still require basic meeting skills to make consultation effective.

Managers must avoid the trap of giving over-long descriptions and justifications of company policy, but rather adopt a more informal question and answer approach. They should try to involve supervisors in giving progress reports on the department rather than doing it all themselves. When there are arguments, managers should avoid becoming the focal point of the debate but encourage group members to discuss issues around the table, instead of directing all the conversation at 'the chair'.

The most important consultative skills are willingness to listen to others, ability to understand their difficulties and to find merit in other peoples' ideas. These can be achieved in practice by summarising the main points someone makes before giving your opinion. This will ensure that understanding is achieved, and will guard against hasty, ill-tempered or destructive reactions. There is a tendency in many people to look for faults and problems in other peoples' bright ideas.

In a consultative meeting the senior nurse should encourage a constructive approach by asking others to put up ideas and suggestions rather than just complaints and criticism. When others accept the invitation, a positive response is to look for the good points in suggestions and express difficulties in a problem-solving way — 'How can we do that in the time available?', not 'We haven't got time.'

Decision-making meetings

We have explained the techniques available to individual managers in making decisions in Chapter 6. These are concerned with adopting some logical strategy for decision-taking and were summarised into 10 phases.

1. Definition of problem
2. Identifying information needed
3. Gathering information
4. Redefining of problem
5. Identification of aims and constraints
6. Finding possible solutions
7. Testing validity of solutions
8. Selecting most appropriate solutions
9. Implementation of decision
10. Follow-up of decision

We observed that there is always a need to involve others in this decision-making process in an appropriate way. Thus, depending on the nature of the problem and the circumstances facing a manager, other people can be asked to assist in all or selected stages of the process.

There are advantages in using a small group to make decisions as well as obvious drawbacks. The potential advantages are:

1. By obtaining several interpretations of a

problem a more acceptable definition can be obtained.

2. There are more sources of information available.
3. Several heads are likely to be better than one in thinking up ideas to solve a problem and considering the practical consequences of adopting them.
4. If individuals are likely to be affected by the outcome of a decision they are more likely to be committed to it if they have been involved in making the decision.

As leader of a group decision-making meeting it is necessary to have clear authority to make decisions in the areas to be discussed. It is also necessary to consider whether decisions will be taken by the leader after consultation or whether they will be truly group decisions emerging out of a concensus. Considerable skills are needed to lead a group through a concensus decision-making process. In the main, they involve introducing the background information, concern and analysis of a problem to the group, then moving the group through the 10 stages of the decision-making process. It is vital that all participants share the same definition of the problem if a genuine group solution is to be achieved. With this shared understanding it may be necessary to adjourn a meeting if essential information is not available.

The great potential benefit of using a group to generate more and better possible solutions will only be realised if the group leader is able to encourage creative thinking. Unfortunately, there are often several elements in management meetings which can inhibit the production of constructive ideas. Some of the most common causes of poor group decision-making and low creativity are:

— The group discussions do not follow a logical decision-making path.
— Time pressures prevent real consideration of a problem.
— A few individuals over-dominate the meeting.
— There is destructive competition between some group members.

— The meeting is too large for real group activity.
— The meeting is run in too formal a style.
— Individuals are inhibited from original suggestions by fear of ridicule.
— The leader does not encourage open discussion and expression of differences.

In response to these common phenomena in group meetings, some techniques have been developed for the purpose of encouraging constructive behaviour and creative thinking. Two of the most useful are called brainstorming and synectics.

Brainstorming

This is an approach to running a complete meeting or to use for a few minutes during a more conventional meeting. The rules are intended to counteract many of the negative aspects of normal encounters outlined above, but particularly the tendency to criticise new ideas without giving them due and open-minded consideration. The main features of a brainstorming meeting are:

1. A group of 4 to 15 can be specially convened to work on a selected problem.
2. The group should be of a mixed membership to deliberately include 'non-experts' who may not be inhibited by over-familiarity with a problem, by conventional wisdom or by established practices.
3. The group leader is responsible for keeping the group to the rules. Thus she is best restricted to being 'process controller'.
4. The group leader, or individual who is most familiar with the problem, explains the background and the type of help required.
5. The leader asks group members for any ideas or suggestions that might seem useful in solving the problem.
6. Ideas should be spontaneously expressed. Ideas need not be obviously practical, they can be funny or apparently far-fetched.
7. The leader records ideas on paper for all to see, so that no ideas are lost.

8. Group members are not allowed to criticise or reject ideas at this stage. Detailed questioning and discussion are also discouraged.
9. The brainstorming session has a set target of producing a number of ideas, or a set time limit.
10. If the meeting is specially arranged as brainstorming, the 'problem owner' can either use the group for further discussion on how some particular ideas could be implemented, or can take the ideas away for later selection and refinement.

If the brainstorming technique has been used in a conventional group meeting to create more possible solutions then the leader can make the group work through the remaining stages of a decision-making process.

Synectics

This technique is a development from brainstorming with similar objectives. It should be used when conventional discussion and investigations of a problem have failed to produce a satisfactory answer. It differs from brainstorming in that it is a more involved process and the intention is to work on selected ideas until the problem owner thinks there is possible practical application and is prepared to commit himself to some action after the meeting. The main features of basic synectics meetings are:

1. Requires a small group with mixed membership and not too many 'experts'.
2. The group leader acts as 'process facilitator'.
3. The person with the problem gives background information to the group and asks for help which is summarised in a sentence beginning 'How to . . . . .'.
4. The leader writes this on a large sheet of paper for the group to see.
5. Group members are asked for spontaneous suggestions on solutions to the problem which are expressed in sentences beginning 'How to . . . . .'.
6. No criticism of suggestions is allowed.

7. Only limited questioning to understand suggestions is allowed.
8. All suggestions are written on sheets of paper by the leader as sentences beginning 'How to . . . . .'.
9. When a reasonable number of suggestions has been obtained the leader asks the 'problem owner' to select one as a possible solution.
10. The problem owner has to say what he likes about the idea. If there are any problems these must be expressed in 'How to . . . . .' sentences.
11. The group then makes further suggestions to overcome these problems.
12. The problem owner is asked by the leader to give feedback of suggestions to show that they are understood, to give positive responses 'What I like about the idea . . . . .' and to express any further difficulties in positive 'How to . . . . .' sentences.
13. The group members are encouraged to build on each others' ideas to find a solution that will overcome the difficulties.
14. The process continues until the problem owner thinks the solution is practical.
15. The group leader asks the problem owner to identify the next step he will take to implement the solution.
16. The process can continue until several possible solutions have been identified.

There are several elaborations on the basic synectics meeting. (See references at the end of this chapter.)

Negotiation meetings

Where there are differences of values, interests, aims or opinions, either between managers or between managers and their staff, it is necessary to resolve these if the organisation is to run smoothly.

There are many circumstances where conflict affects nurse managers, such as in allocation of resources, use of learners, services provided by ancillary staff or the requirement of various medical staff.

Resolving such problems can either be approached by an individual of sufficient authority, power or influence, instructing the disagreeing parties on the way that they will behave, or, more commonly, and usually more satisfactorily, the problem has to be overcome by the process of communication and compromise — negotiation. Thus negotiation meetings are not confined to wage bargaining but to agreeing the terms of a contract between a health authority and an outside supplier. With varying degrees of informality, negotiation is a feature in the nurse manager's job, if we regard negotiation as the means of sorting out disagreement by mutual agreement between those in conflict.

As leader in a negotiation meeting there are two possible roles available. One is to act as an independent mediator between the conflicting parties. The other is to be the 'chief negotiator', pushing your own, or your section's, interest but seeking to find suitable grounds for compromise with the other negotiators. The second role is the most common one for managers.

We give detailed discussion of the broad issues involved in managing conflict in Chapter 16; here we present the main points to observe in conducting a negotiation meeting to resolve issues as a nurse manager either at ward or hospital level. Although preparation is important for all meetings, it is vital in negotiation. You cannot resolve a disagreement without understanding the causes. Thus preliminary consultation and informal discussion is useful both with 'the other side' as well as with your own 'side'. Before attempting negotiation, it is important to be certain you have enough information about the issues and that it is reliable.

At this point it is useful to consider the strengths of your position. The ability to achieve an agreement with others is partly the outcome of power and partly the use of negotiation skills.

Power can come from being in a more senior position than others in a dispute — director of nursing services compared to ward

sister — but this is not the only source of power in work. Having support of a group, or backing of influential individuals, or being the representative of a significant number of junior staff, will give considerable positional power to an individual who occupies an apparently lowly-place in the official hierarchy. A NUPE shop steward may be a porter, but in a negotiation, if he has really got the backing of a significant number of ancillary staff, he may have more power than a general manager. Another source of power can be special knowledge. Thus a sister could have wider experience and understanding of a particular matter than senior nurses, thus giving her considerable 'expert' power to be used in influencing the progress of a negotiation.

Alternatively power can be attached to being in control of essential resources or parts of a process. A ward orderly in a unit which is understaffed may be more crucial to the provision of patient services than a personnel officer, and thus be able to exercise considerable influence in a discussion of problems. Staff in computer departments or maintenance often have considerable 'resource' power.

Thus, before negotiating it is useful to consider several basic questions:

— What is my real power, if any, in this situation?
— What power do others have?
— What do I want ideally?
— What are others likely to want?
— Where are the common interests and areas of likely compromise?
— What are the strengths of my arguments?
— What are their counter-arguments?
— What is the worst possible outcome in the meeting?
— What is my fall-back position — minimum acceptable solution?
— If no agreement can be reached what can we do next?

(There is a choice of admitting failure to agree and retaining existing arrangements, seeking further meetings, referring the matter for conciliation or arbitration to higher authority or taking some direct action.)

— What information should I give before meeting?
— What information should I have available to present at the meeting?
— Can I influence the power base of others by canvassing support for my case?

If two or more people are trying to collaborate on one side of a negotiation meeting, these questions should be discussed between them before the event. They should also agree a teamwork arrangement in which either only one conducts their negotiation, or they have agreed roles. Preparation should also clarify the overall strategy and style to be employed. The main choice in negotiation strategy lies between three alternatives:

1. Make a direct statement of what you want and why you want it, with a clear indication of your power base.
2. Make an overstatement of what you want with the reasons, and an overstatement of the consequences of your not obtaining this outcome. The expectation would be that you are prepared to compromise from this opening stand.
3. Seek to understand the other side's view and demands or possible offers without giving an indication of your own position.

There is no generally correct strategy; the choice will be influenced by existing relationships, the nature of the issue, and the distribution of power. The first approach has the virtue of being unambiguous, but has the potential to lead to deadlock if there is really no room for compromise should the other side refuse to concede. The second approach is used in traditional bargaining over wages, conditions or in buying and selling. It has the virtue of compromise but the disadvantage of deceit and game-playing when applied to more routine situations. The third approach is safest and is particularly relevant where others are seeking changes or making demands. It gives a negotiating advantage if you know

what is in others' hands without disclosing your own.

It is necessary to try to test this to see whether this is their real position or an overstatement on which they are prepared to compromise.

Thus negotiation, involving bargaining and compromise to reach solutions to conflict problems, does involve some game playing. There is a danger of participants getting so involved in the process of negotiation and the wish 'to win' that they lose sight of the main purpose which is to make agreements that are mutually acceptable, workable in practice and will make a contribution to satisfactory health care.

Given sufficient preparation and an appropriate constructive outlook the conduct of a negotiation meeting is similar to that of leading other meetings. A format which can be applied if you wish to control the progress of negotiation is:

1. Open with clarification of purpose and state whether there is authority to make binding decisions on the matter in dispute.
2. Give brief background to the problem and a statement of common interests and common aims.
3. Propose an agenda to discuss the problem. (It can be wise to start with points of least dispute so that early agreements can be made.)
4. Seek a statement from the other side on their views of the problems, proposed solutions, demands and offers.
5. If they are prepared to make this, listen carefully, take notes, ask questions to clarify understanding and test how genuine the statement is.
6. Pick parts of their 'case' where you can agree for discussion and seek agreement.
7. Pick aspects of their 'case' where you have powerful counter-arguments and seek compromise from them.
8. Give your views on the remaining issues, your demands, your offers.

9. Listen to their counter-arguments and proposals.
10. Possibly suggest an adjournment if no agreement has been reached. This will enable both sides to reconsider their position and obtain further information, thus avoiding the danger of deadlock and destructive behaviour.
11. After adjournment, summarise the position (points agreed, points disagreed), seek compromise statement from them, or make compromise offer.
12. If agreement is reached, summarise to be certain that it is really an agreement, make notes on the main points and what action has been agreed.

Some of the key skills required to be an effective negotiator are the willingness to listen and the ability to remain calm even when others are becoming heated. It is better to avoid personal abuse and destructive remarks, the disagreement should be confined to the issues, not personal dislikes. It is useful to summarise what the other side has said, and to seek clarification of any offers or demands made. This helps to keep the atmosphere calm, ensures clear communication and gives thinking time to avoid instant, and later regretted, responses. Patience, persistence and concentration are three particularly useful attributes for negotiators.

REFERENCES

Grove A 1983 High output management (Chapter on meetings). Souvenir Press, London
Janner G 1986 Janner on meetings. Gower, Aldershot
Prince G 1970 The practice of creativity. Collier Books, New York

Memos
Letters
Notices
Formal report writing
Weaknesses in report writing

12
Written Communication

When they wish to contact other people in work most managers prefer to use the telephone or go directly to talk to an individual. There is much to be said in favour of such rapid and direct contact.

There are occasions, however, when managers will consider that written communication, in the form of an internal memo, notice or report, is the best way of presenting information. There will also be a demand on managers to produce papers for senior management, to write minutes of meetings, and to correspond with the outside world: the more senior the post the more requirement to write; the more advisory the post the more demand for written confirmation.

Thus there is a general need for all nurse managers to develop skills in using the various written communications media. They must be able to produce unambiguous statements that achieve the purpose of the communication quickly.

The main points to observe in business writing are, like the general principles of communication, simple common sense. Having decided that writing is the suitable medium, it is useful to consider a number of points before putting pen to paper or fingers to keyboard, the most important being to clarify the purpose. There are several distinct objectives in writing:

— To inform readers about a particular topic
— To inform and request advice or information about a topic

— To inform and influence the opinions of readers
— To pass on specific instructions
— To inform and make recommendations on a particular course of action.

The structure, content and style of a written message should be consistent with the main purpose. In deciding how to structure and write a particular piece, a manager can usefully ask four questions:

1. Who are the intended reader/readers?
2. What is their existing knowledge of the topic?
3. What are their attitudes towards the topic and the writer?
4. What are the important points of the message?

In producing simple minutes after a health care team meeting there may be two sets of readers with different needs. Those who attended the meeting and those who did not but are interested in the outcome. The first group will require only a brief action sheet simply listing points agreed and who will take actions by what particular date. The second may need more background information on topics discussed at the meeting.

To produce a simple paper for a unit general manager recommending the purchase of new equipment for the unit, the writer should consider the existing medical knowledge of the GM, costs involved, the current policy towards expenditure and the benefits to patients. This will indicate how much background information is needed and how the benefits of purchase can be best sold to the GM.

Such preliminary thought will usually save time if it means that the piece need only be written once. For a simple memo, letter or notice it may be possible to keep the overall structure in mind whilst actually writing. For longer papers, reports, articles, etc, it is better to write out the structure as a series of headings. These can then be placed in a logical order.

A document with a simple, logical structure will be easy to read. Clarity of thought leads to clarity of expression. There are several ways to arrange information in management documents. The most common is:

Title or heading	This is essential for every management document.
Introduction	This may be one sentence which gets the matter underway.
Aim	Clear statement of the purpose of a report, letter, memo: why it was written, what it covers, order in which material is covered.
Main content	Facts, opinions, appraisal of the issues.
Conclusions	Logical outcome of the arguments and facts.
Recommendation	Clear indication of action (or non-action) emerging from conclusions.
Summary	If the document is long or complex a brief statement of contents will be useful. This can then be placed at the beginning.

Within this framework it will be necessary to structure the 'main content' logically. This can be done in several ways:

1. Chronological sequence of events or issues (start at the beginning and work forward).
2. Statement in summary of a problem.
   Analysis of the problem in detail.
   Outline of possible solutions.
3. Outline of a proposal or proposition.
   Evidence supporting this.
4. Proposal for action.
   Summary of the need for such action.
   Outline of possible outcomes from the action.
   Expected benefits from the action.

In longer documents clarity is helped by using headings and sub-headings. It is common to number sections. This can be done by labelling main headings 1, 2, 3, 4 etc.

and subsections (a), (b), (c), or (i), (ii), (iii). Another convention in reports is to number sub-sections in a decimal form — 1.1, 1.2, 1.3., 2.1, 2.2, 2.3 etc.

The choice of style (words used, tone, length of paragraphs, etc.) should also be consistent with the purpose and readership. If the piece is important then it will usually benefit from being rewritten, edited and polished two or even three times. In this case, use the framework as a guide, and set time aside in a quiet place to write a rough draft quickly in one sitting. Do not seek for perfection at this stage. Write furiously in pace with your thoughts. It is useful to type in double or treble space or to handwrite on alternate lines on one side of the paper. This makes later rewriting and changes of the structure easy.

If time allows, this first draft should be put to one side. Some hours or a day later, re-read the whole in one sitting to check the logic of the structure (would point three be better before point two, etc?), and improve the style by rewriting and polishing the first effort. The aim in all management writing should be to use direct, simple language which presents information as clearly as possible. George Orwell recommended a formula for writing straightforward text that has become widely adopted:

1. Never use a metaphor, simile or other figure of speech which you are used to seeing in print.
2. Never use a long word where a short word will do.
3. If it is possible to cut out a word, always cut it out.
4. Never use the passive where you can use the active.
5. Never use a foreign phrase, a scientific word or a jargon word if you can think of an everyday English equivalent.
6. Break any of these rules sooner than say anything barbarous.

For business writing, points 2,3 and 4 are of greatest significance. Make each sentence contain one idea or fact only. This will make sentences short and quick to read. Similarly, new paragraphs should be used for each new topic or aspect of the subject.

In the revision of a document, remove unnecessary words, break up long sentences and paragraphs, check for spelling mistakes, rewrite clumsy phrases and correct obvious grammatical errors.

Although the use of jargon should be discouraged in external communication, there is a specialised language which professionals or members of the same organisation share. Thus it is quicker to use such language, but only if it is really understood by the reader.

These guidelines are applicable to all document writing. There are some more specific points to consider in some specialised forms of management writing, such as memos, letters, notices, reports. Although it is likely that most senior staff in nursing will be familiar with the purpose and convention attached to these particular forms of written communication, we have provided brief guidance in order to give a comprehensive cover of this topic.

Memos

These are internal communications usually between people who are known to each other. They should be written in a brief and direct style with the minimum of formalities. As an internal note, memos can be handwritten or typed; answers can be added by the receiver to save time although it may be advisable to retain a copy of memos and replies. A common format is shown below:

INTERNAL MEMO

FROM	TO
POSITION	POSITION
TEL	DATE
	SUBJECT:

Letters

Letters are generally used for external communication. Each letter as an official message from a representative of an organisation is usually required to follow the 'house' form and style of the organisation. Usually a letter deals with one subject only.

In writing business letters there are several conventions to observe:

1. Letters usually contain a reference number of figures indicating the author's initials and a filing number.
2. Letters should start with a heading or title.
3. Letters usually show the full address and name of the recipient.
4. Letters usually start with the reason for writing.
   (In reply to your letter of . . .; as agreed at our meeting of . . .: I understand you are interested in. . ., etc.)

There are also some practical considerations in composing letters:

1. Think about the content of a letter before writing.
2. Possibly note headings of main points to be covered.
3. Try to write, or dictate, to get the letter right in one attempt.
4. Using standard phrases, paragraphs or whole letters will save time.

Notices

A notice for display on the internal board or other public place needs to meet certain requirements.

1. The content should be brief, direct and unambiguous.
2. The words used should be simple. Sentences should be short.
3. It must contain an eye catching title or heading.
4. It must indicate who was the originator and show their authority.
5. It should be typed or printed clearly, with headings using colour or illustrations to attract attention.

Formal report writing

There is sometimes a need for nurse managers to produce more extensive documents in the style of formal reports. Although there is benefit in writing in a comprehensive way, there is a tendency for managers and professional staff in large bureaucracies to write at length instead of using briefer and more direct means of communication. As a result, many managers at all levels feel overwhelmed by the volume of paper which arrives on their desks.

Thus before commissioning or writing a report, it is essential to have identified that it is needed and is the most appropriate medium for communication. The main purposes in producing a report will be:

1. To provide information and updating on progress, plans, technical and clinical developments, professional innovations and organisational issues. or
2. To provide information and analysis of a major problem with conclusions, possible solutions or recommendations as an aid to decision-making by those with appropriate authority.

Thus documents can be prepared by junior staff for submission to more senior staff; by managers for consideration by a group of colleagues or their own staff team; by senior managers as information, advice or instruction for more junior staff.

If the report has been commissioned, it is essential to obtain detailed briefing to be clear on the precise purpose, deadline, authority and resources available, final form required and any interim reporting.

A conventional structure to follow in management and professional reports is:

Title:	What is the paper called?
Prepared by:	Who has written it?
Intended for:	Who are the readers?
Contents page:	If a long report.
Introduction:	What is the paper about?
	Why has it been written?
	What are the terms of reference?

Background and history:

Description of events, situation, summary of problem etc., to enable reader to appreciate the background.

Analysis of the problem: or summary of progress, achievement, outcome of action:

If the paper is intended to draw attention to a difficulty which needs resolution, the main symptoms and possible causes of the problem need to be described.

If the paper is a record of actions that have been undertaken, these need to be described with the outcomes.

Possible solutions:

If a problem has been analysed, the choices of action to resolve it can be outlined.

Conclusions:

A summary of either the main issues still to be resolved in a problem or the level of success achieved by the course of action.

Recommendations:

If appropriate, a course of future action can be suggested.

Summary:

The main points covered can be briefly summarised. It can be useful to place this summary at the beginning of the paper.

Appendices:

In order to reduce the content of the main report it is useful to include background material and detailed information in a separate section at the end.

Weaknesses in report writing

Many reports fail to achieve either the purpose of conveying information in a usable form or in persuading others to accept the recommendations. The main weaknesses in poor reports are:

1. Structure does not follow a logical sequence or the structure is not clearly described at the beginning.
2. Insufficient or unclear description of the background of a problem (too much is assumed of the reader).
3. Description of a problem and recommendations are mixed together.
4. Too much information is presented without the writer identifying the key issues and the main trends.
5. There is no clear 'main theme' to the paper.
6. Main arguments are not supported with factual information or do not take account of all issues involved.
7. Recommendations do not demonstrate clearly why they are the preferred solutions.
8. Conclusions and recommendations do not follow logically from the analysis, or there is a failure to present any in a precise form.
9. Recommendations are not based on a 'cost benefit analysis', but on generalised declarations that the action would be desirable.
10. Recommendations do not indicate precisely how they are to be put into practice.

REFERENCES

Chappell R T, Read W L 1979 Business communication. MacDonald and Evans, Plymouth
Padget P 1983 Communication and reports. Cassell, London

13

Managers and motivation

Providing health care is a team activity. Senior management needs to create organisational structures and relationships that foster collaboration between staff in all parts of a health service. Individual nurse managers should develop constructive relationships within their own unit, as well as with senior nurses, medical, administrative, ancillary and unit management staff, who in turn should co-operate with each other. A few managers have the right combination of knowledge, natural communication skills and personal charisma that enable them to maintain satisfactory relationships throughout this network. Most managers have to work hard in developing and maintaining relationships which often fall below the ideal of a collaborative team.

Given that nurses receive professional training which includes a study of human behaviour, and that nurses spend time dealing with people under stress, the human aspects of management should not present great difficulties.

There can be significant differences in the relationship between a nurse and a patient/client, where the aim is caring and helping, and the relationship between senior nurse and nurses, where the aim is to provide appropriate leadership so that work targets are achieved. Even more difficult for many nurse managers is the task of working in partnership with doctors and general managers.

All nurse managers need to be aware of the general theories concerning behaviour in work and the various prescriptions that are put forward on how relationships in work can be managed effectively. In addition, managers need to develop insights about their own motivations in work, personality character- istics, values and attitudes. Being self-aware means you can be sensitive to others. You should understand your own behaviour, the effect of your impact on others and the poss- ible causes of their behaviour. The skills of inter-personal communication discussed in Chapter 9 are relevant and central to this aim.

MOTIVATION AND WORK

Everyone who is employed in health care needs a combination of knowledge and the will to use knowledge consistently in positive and responsible ways. It is not clear as to what comes first, knowledge or motivation. To acquire professional qualifications and prac- tical skills to be a competent staff nurse requires motivation, yet there are trained and knowledgeable staff who are unable to apply this fully or consistently in their jobs. Clearly, these are complementary qualities. Motivation without knowledge is possibly more dangerous than knowledge without motivation, but the absence of either is a major problem.

This condition applies equally to learner nurses, ward auxiliaries, porters, sisters and senior nurse managers. Where does positive motivation to work come from? Does it come from individuals themselves, or do we have to be motivated by others?

All human beings have motivation — conscious needs and goals for which individ- uals are prepared to expend energy and skill. There are also a number of unconscious aspects of personality which push the indi- vidual into activity. We all have some choice in how we spend our time, how we earn our living and how we behave in various situations life presents. Without motivation we would be passive, exercise no choice and show no individuality. Everyone with practical experi- ence in work can identify significant differ- ences in the way individuals behave and

differences between the behaviour of different groups.

Logically, the ideal organisation should start by selecting staff with appropriate motivation. In reality this is unlikely to be possible. There are few occasions when organisations are built from scratch, and even when new staff are recruited it is very difficult to assess their motivation. It is easier to assess an applicant's qualifications and previous experience. Even individuals who have shown admirable quali- ties in previous jobs, do not always behave similarly with their next employer.

It is clear that the extent to which someone displays positive motivation is the result of how their basic qualities (intelligence, person- ality, attitudes, values and skills), their expec- tations of their particular employment, their current needs and goals combine with the circumstance of a particular job.

Thus while it is sensible management policy to aim at recruiting staff with good potential, it is just as important to ensure that the circumstances of employment will have a positive effect on their motivation.

In many organisations, both in health care and elsewhere, this is a mammoth and, some would suggest, an impossible task. There is a view that morale of many staff in the NHS declined in the 1970s and 80s as a result of re- organisation, shortage of resources and a history of inconsiderate management. Such morale problems do not automatically mean that individuals will not do their best to provide patient care, but if their motivation to do a professional job has diminished it is very difficult to reverse the process. Attitudes of dissatisfaction may mean staff become more hostile towards higher management, resistant to efforts aimed at changing administration systems, and experience increased stress from caring for others while working in an organ- isation that does not seem to care for them.

While some senior nurses may share this criticism of their health authority, by accepting posts of responsibility, they should take a lead in motivating themselves and others to apply their best endeavours in their sphere of influ- ence, whatever the problems.

The basic and simple assumption underlying the various theories which have been put forward in an attempt to explain the behaviour of people in work is that man willingly expends energy if by doing so he expects to receive a reward. The more difficult questions that emerge from this obvious principle for managers in nursing are:

— What are the rewards which might motivate health service staff?
— Are these within the control of nurse managers?
— How can a clear link between good job performance and reward be established by managers?

REWARDS IN WORK

Rewards can be tangible (figures on a wage slip, a clear desk, a patient being discharged) or less tangible (a smile from a patient, praise from a ward sister), features of work which an individual feels pleased to receive. Although individuals differ in what they expect from work, motivation theories suggest that human beings are affected by the same basic needs. Most managers who undertake formal study of behaviour in work are presented with some widely known theories based on the writing of a psychologist, A. Maslow (1943). He has put forward a framework of human motivation in which these common needs are ranked in hierarchical order. These are:

1. Physical or physiological needs (for food, warmth, shelter, etc.)
2. Safety or security needs
3. Love needs (for community, companionship or the affection of others)
4. Need for self-esteem (to have a high regard of your own worth), and
5. Need for self-actualisation (using your potential and becoming all you are capable of becoming).

The theory suggests that for a fully satisfactory life you require satisfaction of all your needs. In modern Western society the lower needs are generally provided, so the motivation of mature adults is directed towards satisfaction of the higher needs.

An extension of this theory has been made by another often quoted American, F. Herzberg (1966). He relates this hierarchy of needs to work in describing two sets of conditions in work. One he terms the 'Hygiene' factors which he uses to describe aspects of work necessary to satisfy the lower needs — pay, working environment, facilities, welfare policies, etc. He regards these as causes for dissatisfaction and suggests that management has to provide conditions which will remove motivation blocks, but these alone will not provide positive satisfaction in work. This depends upon the factors he calls 'motivators', which can be a source of positive satisfaction in work. These are a sense of achievement, recognition, intrinsic interest in job tasks, responsibility and advancement.

One conclusion from such a view of human motivation and work in large organisations is that management should develop a system that enables staff to contribute to the goals of the organisation by doing jobs which provide scope for individual satisfaction, rather than break work into simple and repetitive tasks which are closely supervised, only offering financial compensation. This implies that individuals should be encouraged to take responsibility for planning and monitoring their own work, that jobs should contain enough variety and challenge to provide a sense of achievement. This process has been called 'job enrichment'.

Many managers consider this to be an idealistic and impractical concept. They expect that financial reward and fears of reprimand or possible dismissal, together with good working environments, close control and adequate communication, will ensure that staff work to standards. Another frequently quoted authority on motivation has described managers who hold this view as perpetuating an instrumental or 'Theory X' concept and those managers with a more humanistic outlook as 'Theory Y', (McGregor 1960).

Although these theorists are American and

were mainly concerned with management and motivation in commercial enterprises, they provide a useful framework for British managers in public sector organisations to reflect on their particular motivation problems. Nurse managers, whether employed in the NHS or in private health care, should consider the potential rewards in their own work, and that of their own staff, their colleagues and more senior staff, and how these influence motivation and behaviour.

A list of factors which will be relevant for such an analysis by senior nurses can be grouped together as the potential rewards from work under six headings related to the hierarchy of needs:

1. Financial rewards. The material benefits from employment obtained from basic pay, overtime allowances, subsidised meals, subsidised accommodation, allowances, etc.
2. Security rewards. The feeling of security from a dependable level of earnings, continuity of employment, assurances of future employment, transferable skills.
3. Social rewards. The involvement with others, being a member of a team, being part of a community.
4. Status and recognition rewards. Membership of a 'profession' or skilled group, held in high regard by professional colleagues, high regard of patients/clients, praise from more senior staff, involvement in decisions, power, position in a hierarchy.
5. Advancement rewards. Prospects of promotion, career structure with higher pay in higher grades.
6. Achievement rewards. Sense of fulfilment and self-actualisation by using skills, opportunities to learn, variety in work tasks, interest in work tasks, interest in medicine, belief in caring values, tangible outcome from personal efforts, some autonomy, exercising discretion.

Financial rewards

The pay and other economic benefits from work are a significant factor in deciding to change jobs, or, for some people, when selecting a particular occupation. Pay is also a significant source of dissatisfaction, usually as a result of comparisons.

If you feel that others using a similar amount of skill and effort (or less) or with similar (or fewer) responsibilities earn more than you do, this will be a source of resentment. These comparisons can be made both with others working for the same organisation, or with those working elsewhere. Thus for many people pay is not a motivational factor, it is simply a requirement to get someone to take a job and is regarded as a right; or it is a source of demotivation if it is perceived as being basically inadequate or inequitable.

For pay to be a positive factor in motivating staff to work effectively, there has to be a direct link between job performance and financial reward. Systems of 'payment by results' or bonus schemes are designed to make this connection. There is usually an increase in output under such schemes but, unless carefully monitored, there can be lower quality work and reduced flexibility amongst staff. It has been observed that incentive schemes tend to have a diminishing effect unless they are reviewed regularly.

Another system that tries to make pay a direct motivator is that of individual merit awards. Staff performance is assessed regularly and pay increases awarded according to merit. The potential motivational advantages have to be weighed against the practical problems of assessing individual worth fairly and the dangers of demotivating staff who feel that favouritism is the major influence in awarding merit increases.

A number of incentive payment schemes have been introduced into the NHS for various support and ancillary workers. In the case of nurses and others involved in direct patient care, it seems inappropriate to use 'payment by results' or merit payment schemes. Pay, however, is an important issue for nurses, but has generally been a source of dissatisfaction. In one study of nursing staff in a mental hospital (Clark 1978) half the male nurses and a quarter of the females stated that pay was the most important reward they expected from work. Many complained about the low level of pay, yet only 5 out of 75 stated that they were dissatisfied with their job as a whole. In choosing nursing as an occupation, 40% were influenced by a basic interest in helping people and 60% influenced by practical reasons such as locality, shortage of other work or a need for professional qualifications.

Security

A feeling of security can be an outcome of the particular relationship between individuals and their working environment. If you are familiar with the tasks, problems and pressures in a particular job and have regularly been able to cope with them, you will feel confident and psychologically secure. You also need some economic security from assurance that your actual employment will be reasonably stable, that your earnings will not be subject to unreasonable fluctuations and that you will not suffer from arbitrary discipline and dismissal.

Where management provides adequate training, gives appropriate advice, communicates effectively and offers proper support to staff, this will do much to induce the necessary psychological stability to work. Where management is able to plan for the successful continuation of an organisation and develops personnel policies, giving assurances of no compulsory redundancy, most staff could also be expected to feel reasonably secure in the economic aspects.

Staff will seek ways of increasing their own sense of security. This can manifest itself in a reluctance to change traditional methods of working and adopting restrictive or protective practices at work.

Feelings of insecurity can also lead to disruptive behaviour, lack of co-operation and the belief in rumours.

Thus at corporate level, appropriate personnel policies and procedures have to be created to meet these basic economic security needs. At a unit level, although individual nurse managers can do little about the economic factors of work, they can do much to provide support that will encourage feelings of psychological security. We consider the means for achieving this in the sections in this chapter on Leadership style and Handling stress.

Social rewards

It is inevitable that when people work together they will not simply be a collection of individuals but will form a social system. Part of this system is made from the official structure of an organisation in that people are in sections and teams with official targets, procedures and relationships. There is a significant informal social system in existence as well. Team members develop their own way of carrying out their duties; they may develop an unofficial hierarchy and a code of conduct. New members of staff soon become aware of these 'tribal' customs and realise that they need to conform if they are to be accepted by their fellow workers. Membership of an official work team and the variety of informal relationships in work are a substantial attraction and compensation for many of us in work. (One of the unhappy consequences of unemployment is a feeling of being outside the working community and the loss of companionship.)

This phenomenon is both a benefit and a challenge to managers. Work groups can be self-motivating and self-controlled, thus ensuring that individual members maintain a proper level of work output and quality. Such forces can assist managers by removing the need for constant supervision and guidance. Some managers also find such group pressures a threat. They feel that they are not fully in control of a situation and that the standard maintained by a group is not consistent with the objectives of management. A ward sister who is appointed from outside a unit sometimes finds on arrival that clinical practices and staffing arrangements which have been established for some time are unacceptable.

This can create conflict which takes time and skill to resolve.

Clearly, the aim of managers should be to ensure that the social rewards and the informal social system of work groups are consistent with the organisational aims, not a source of disruption.

This can be achieved by encouraging individual members to co-operate and help each other with their work tasks and to regard the work and success of a unit as a collective responsibility, not that of the unit supervisor alone. Attention should be given to communication and involving staff so that they are committed to achieving high standards. Then encouragement can be given to flexibility, open communication and informality. Feelings of being valued members of a team should be given to all unit members.

Although health care has been officially organised into health care teams, multidisciplinary teams and nursing teams, there have been complaints by NHS staff of the continuation of authoritarian and insular attitudes by some medical, nursing and administrative staff, which undermines the creation of really co-operative team work.

The Powys Health Authority has recognised this problem, and at some hospitals has not only broken down the barriers that often exist between community nurses and hospital nurses by making them into an integrated nursing team, but has also involved ambulance drivers, clerical workers, porters and other staff whose work is an indispensable part of health care provision. We consider this further in the sections on leadership style and team building.

Status and recognition

We all need to hold ourselves in high regard, to feel we have worth as an individual. For most individuals self-respect is enhanced by or even depends upon the relationship with others for whom we have respect, both in work and in our lives outside.

Being employed to work for and alongside other people offers potential rewards to our recognition needs, as well as many threats to our ego. Membership of a recognised profession, generally held in high regard, is another source of satisfaction. Acceptance by our peers as a worthwhile member of a work group is another. Praise from those who supervise our work, or who are at the receiving end, is a further source of reward.

'To come into hospital and work with people and learn more about yourself and learn to be more understanding . . . it's very rewarding.' — nursing assistant

(quoted by Clark, 1978)

Working as a nurse should offer satisfaction of recognition needs by receiving praise and gratitude from patients, respect from fellow health care workers and support from senior professional colleagues. Unfortunately, not all nurses work in such satisfactory environments, and may find the stress involved in providing patient care, relative isolation from helpful colleagues, reliance on trainee or temporary staff and insensitivity of medical staff can make theirs a thankless task.

Although it should always be a major part of a nurse manager's role to provide nursing staff with proper recognition, it is particularly so when this is lacking from other quarters. Unfortunately, some senior nurses not only fail to fulfil this requirement but can even undermine the recognition needs of others by accentuating their own status through excessive formality, emphasis on discipline and using an authoritarian manner.

Mary Clark concluded from her study of nursing staff's motivations that most were 'dissatisfied with the amount of influence they had and were dissatisfied with the status they had'.

It is equally important to be sensitive to the needs of staff who work in jobs that are not accorded a very high status in the organisational structure. In the NHS there have been complaints by so called auxiliary nurses and ancillary workers (this title could imply that they are non-essential and therefore of lower status) that they are not really regarded as members of the health care team to be accorded respect by the more professionally qualified staff.

In the sections on leadership and team building in Chapter 13 we give further consideration of how nurse managers can adopt a style in relationships with others that takes account of this basic need for recognition and status.

Achievement

Most people look for greater purpose in working than simply the pay packet it provides. There is a need to feel that your work has some intrinsic significance.

Such a sense of achievement is a reward which can emerge from several aspects of employment. There may be a belief in the overall purpose of the organisation for which you work, or the overall value of what you have to do each day. Clearly, many people in all health care occupations have a fundamental conviction that caring for the sick is essential and worthwhile. Many will feel that their personal role plays a direct and important part in helping individual patients. Naturally there are also health workers who appear to be less interested in this caring aspect.

Having an overall identification with the purpose of your work will not in isolation ensure a sense of achievement. Indeed, it can create problems, as a firm conviction and dedication to a cause can lead you to suffer greater frustrations and stress when events do not coincide with your conceptions.

A positive sense of achievement will emerge when you feel that the tasks you perform each day produce tangible and worthwhile results. If, in addition, these tasks require you to exercise skills that you value, to use your judgements within your capacity, are varied enough to maintain your interest and fill each day but without excessive demand, these will be the main components of job satisfaction from a sense of purpose and achievement.

There are several possible combinations of these elements. It is possible to find a job with sufficient challenge, interest and variety to give a sense of achievement, but without believing in the ultimate product or purpose of your organisation (Medical Officer in cigarette manufacturing; Army Chaplain, etc.). It is possible to work in an organisation in which you believe but where your actual job provides little intrinsic satisfaction. The extreme is unsatisfactory work in an organisation you dislike, and the ideal is a fulfilling job in a worthwhile organisation.

The general intrinsic factors which can be manipulated by managers to increase the potential of a job to meet achievement needs can be summarised as:

1. Having specific goals or targets which are demanding of your particular skills but attainable (both individually and as a member of a work team)
2. Obtaining direct feedback on the outcome of your efforts that is either self-evident (drugs round completed, paperwork cleared away, etc.) or comes from others (evaluation questionnaires, colleague reactions, senior manager's praise)
3. Being able to use a range of skills which you value and which you believe are usefully applied
4. Having some freedom to organise your work and to exercise personal judgement
5. Having some variety in the tasks you have to do
6. Having an opportunity to acquire greater knowledge and skills, and to contribute to the learning of others
7. To feel that you are becoming more effective in a role.

Managers who wish to enhance the potential sense of achievement for staff will seek regular meetings with them individually and in work teams, to clarify and agree work targets and objectives, to agree improvements and projects, and to give regular feedback on results achieved. Managers should also try to provide data as frequently as possible for staff to assess their own level of achievement. There can also be deliberate attempts by managers to change the design of jobs so that the achievement factors are increased.

There are three ways of approaching this. One is by increasing flexibility between staff and rotating available work tasks more widely. This is intended to increase variety, interest, scope for learning and to enhance promotion prospects. A second approach is that of intentionally building into jobs wider scope and more tasks, instead of specialisation and narrowly defined roles. This is the process of job enlargement. The third seeks to add responsibility so staff do more planning and organisation of their own work, check their own quality and undertake improvements — this is job enrichment.

In health care there are basic differences in the demands and potential rewards to be found in the various nursing roles. A district nurse may experience freedom from close supervision, variety of client and locality, but may also feel isolated and lack immediate feedback of results. A staff nurse in a theatre will be able to use skills, work as a team member and see immediate outcome from completed operations, but will be under direct and close supervision. It is not possible for immediate nurse managers to make fundamental changes in the duties of nursing staff or the division of responsibilities between different parts of the service, but it is possible to try to build in some agreed targets, results, feedback, encouragement, autonomy, variety and learning into the jobs of subordinate staff, according to the various needs of staff, by delegation, coaching, allocation of duties and style of managing. It is possible for senior management in health care to consult with staff about the content of jobs and the allocation of responsibility, with a view to identifying the need for and the possible way of introducing greater job flexibility, job enlargement or job enrichment.

SEEING THINGS AS OTHERS SEE THEM

In this chapter we have tried to present a theory about behaviour in work which is based on the assumption that positive motivation towards our work will be an outcome of what we expect the rewards of work to be and the extent to which these are available in a particular work-place. Some people may be able to adjust to expecting work only to be instrumental in providing the economic means of living. Most people, however, have perceptions that work can also provide social contact, interest, recognition and a sense of purpose.

Not all the reward factors are within the control of nurse managers, however. Clearly, terms and conditions of employment are established at national and corporate level, as are policies concerning issues such as professional training, promotion procedures or redundancy. Local managers are still required to do the best they can in their own work tasks and to have satisfactory unit staff; thus if staff performance is not at a satisfactory level it is their responsibility to consider the possible causes. These are likely to be one or a combination of factors when an individual is not doing a good job:

— Lack of basic ability on their part for the type of work
— Inadequate induction into particular job
— Lack of adequate training or instruction in tasks
— Lack of experience of particular tasks
— Inadequacy of resources or environment
— Dissatisfied with some aspects of job content
— Unsatisfactory organisation of work
— Unsatisfactory leadership from immediate manager
— Unsatisfactory support from other team members
— Dissatisfaction with some aspects of employment
— Temporary personal problems.

To interpret the behaviour of others accurately it is necessary to understand how they see things, to appreciate their point of view and their problems. This can be difficult for a manager who may himself be subject to stress and demotivation. Thus there is a tendency to analyse a situation from a 'should do' standpoint. The staff 'should' appreciate the importance of good quality work . . ., 'should' accept that conditions are reasonable, etc. We behave according to our interpretation of reality not from the way others believe we should interpret it, or from their interpretation. If I find my job boring it is boring to me, even if you think I should find it interesting. Thus managers wishing to influence the behaviour of their staff should be close enough to them to understand their expectations, satisfactions and frustrations.

In talking with staff about their experience of work and monitoring their performance, a sister may identify relatively simple problems in staff needing clearer instructions, more training or clarification of specific procedures. There may be aspects of job content that could be altered to give more or less responsibility and variety. Staff may also indicate some dissatisfaction with the way they believe they are managed by the sister, or with the quality of relationships between unit staff. This can be difficult for a sister to accept. But as managers expect others to take notice of feedback and criticism in order to improve performance, they should be prepared to apply the same process to their own managerial approach. An effective manager is a learning manager, a flexible and adaptable manager.

It is essential to understand all that is involved in managing relationships: the main components can be identified as:

— Leadership and management style
— Team building
— Handling conflict and stress
— Handling problem individuals
— Handling discipline
— Managing change.

Although these issues have been treated separately they should form a consistent and complete concept for the task of managing other people and relationships at work.

REFERENCES

Clark M 1978 Getting through the work. In: Dingwell R, McIntosh J (eds) Readings in the sociology of nursing. Churchill Livingstone, Edinburgh
Handy C 1976 Understanding organisations. Penguin Books, London
Herzberg F 1966 Work and the nature of man, World publishing company,
Maslow A 1943 A theory of human motivation. Psychological Review (New York)
McGregor D 1960 The human side of enterprise. McGraw-Hill, Maidenhead
Stein L 1978 The doctor-nurse game. In: Dingwell R, McIntocsh J (eds) Readings in the sociology of nursing. Churchill Livingstone, Edinburgh
Vroom V, Deci E 1970 Management and motivation. Penguin Books, London

14

Leadership and management style

MANAGEMENT STYLE

A considerable amount of research and training is available to help managers who wish to become more effective leaders, but what does the concept of leadership mean for senior nurses in the NHS or nurse managers in independent health care?

As a section head or team leader they have responsibilities to allocate work, make decisions, introduce changes, and exercise control concerning the work of their units. Thus they need to influence the behaviour of staff in a constructive way. This is a leadership role. The way that a senior nurse approaches this task will be a reflection of her beliefs about the right way to manage staff — this is termed 'management style'

Attempts have been made to identify distinguishable styles used by managers. It is common to define two extremes. One would be typified by an individual who favoured making decisions that affect staff without reference to them and who favoured giving direct instructions. If changes were introduced these would be worked out in detail by the manager before being imposed on staff. This type of manager perceives herself as a separate leader and subordinate staff are expected to accept their role as 'the led'.

The opposite form of management style manifests itself in a manager who passes decision-making down as far as possible, who deliberately involves staff in problems and in planning, and expects development proposals from them. Changes would be implemented after discussion and, ideally, by mutual agreement. This type of manager perceives herself as team leader and staff as full members of the team.

The first style has been called 'autocratic' or 'directive' and the second 'democratic' or 'participative'(Tannembaum & Schmidt 1958)

Theorists in this field have developed frameworks into which it is possible to fit variations between these extremes. A widely-accepted model has a modification of the autocratic style where a manager still seeks to impose decisions, instructions and changes on others, but seeks to court acceptance by staff through explanation and persuasion. This is labelled 'persuasive style'. A modification of the participative approach can be identified where a manager seeks to make decisions, give instructions, and introduce changes, after consideration of staff views and suggestions. This style is called 'consultative', but if this is to be genuine the manager has to be prepared to modify decisions and incorporate staff views into final plans.

There is a tendency to suggest that the consultative approaches are more effective than directive styles. This style is considered more likely to obtain co-operation and commitment from staff and lead them to develop greater competence. This view is clearly consistent with motivation theories which emphasise our need for recognition and achievement. There is also evidence from practical studies of nursing staff attitudes in the NHS, supporting the supposition that staff wish to be more involved in the management processes at ward level (Clark 1978).

Other management researchers (Licket 1961) suggest that managers have two main areas of concern. One is a concern for 'production' (output of work, quality of service, accuracy, etc.), the other is concern for 'people' (seeking satisfaction of human needs, relating to people in a genuine manner rather than only as a means of production). Some managers have an inclination to direct greater energies into one aspect, being either more 'production centred' or more 'people centred'.

Either extreme is considered ineffective. Ironically, the production-centred manager often alienates staff, who then respond with poor productive effort, forcing the management to be even more strictly production centred. The general model for effective management is suggested as one who has a high concern for both 'production' and 'human' factors, 9.9 on the management grid (Blake & Mouton 1978).

There are other opinions (Feilder 1967) about the universal application of consultative or 9.9 management styles. These suggest that some individuals and work groups expect their managers to be directive, and will not respond to a more participative approach. There is also the issue of staff competence; some individuals will be more self-directed, requiring a 'management by exception' control, but will expect to be consulted on issues affecting them. Other staff with less ability or experience will require closer supervision and will have less to contribute to planning or decision-making.

Given these variations and such factors as the technology of work, content of jobs, the culture of the organisation and the limited amount of authority and power held by a manager, there is a school of thought suggesting that managers need to be flexible in their choice of management style. This implies that a manager should assess the particular situation in which she has to operate and choose a style which is the best fit (Hersey & Blanchard 1977). There can be little objection to the logic of this proposition. There may be practical problems, however, for a manager in trying to make a dispassionate assessment of circumstances in which she is directly involved, and doubts on whether individuals can be flexible enough to adopt several different styles. Flexibility may be interpreted as inconsistency — although staff do not like authoritarian management if a manager always acts in this way, they at least know where they stand.

Flexibility may also be considered by others

as indecisiveness. A common complaint about middle and junior management is that they are unable to make decisions, are leaders in name but not in practice. This can be caused by an authoritarian senior nurse with a low regard for ward level supervisors and considerable knowledge about details of ward processes, bypassing and undermining supervisors and so forcing them to abdicate their leadership role to use an 'accommodative' style of management.

The practical conclusion from such theoretical considerations of leadership style is that as a nurse manager you should be aware of your own preferences as a leader and aware of the impact these have on immediate staff. You should also be aware of your senior colleagues' preferences and the impact of their style on you and your staff.

Frank discussion amongst a team can seem threatening, not only to the leader but to members, unless this is part of the organisational culture. Within psychiatric care, open team meetings are more common than in the general hospital service. Some nurse managers may prefer more discreet conversations with individual team members, or wish to use training sessions conducted by an outsider to facilitate a safer examination of group feelings.

As a result of such a review a manager may wish to modify her present approach. It is useful to consider how this intention might be achieved in practice. We include a general list of desirable behaviours for all managers and some further suggestions for those wishing to move towards a more directive or more consultative style.

Generally desirable characteristics for nurse managers

1. Treat all staff as human beings rather than simply the means of completing work tasks. Get to know their backgrounds, interests, expectations, personalities and problems.
2. Be aware of staff difficulties, irritations and complaints. Be seen to take action on these wherever possible. Explain reasons when this is not possible.
3. Be seen to have influence with more senior managers. Prevent other managers from directly intervening in your unit. Stand up for your staff.
4. Be seen to have influence over medical staff. Do not let them treat nurses in an arbitrary or unreasonable way.
5. Be seen to have influence with ancillary and service departments.
6. Look for reason to praise staff. Many managers give little direct feedback except when mistakes are made.
7. When things go wrong, look for positive solutions to overcome difficulties, rather than try to allocate blame.
8. Accept responsibility for everything that happens in your unit.
9. Never belittle others. Show respect to all whatever their level of skill or place in the official hierarchy.
10. Be seen as a helper to staff; give time to counselling those with difficulties.
11. Walk the job regularly to show interest and support for staff and their work, not just to check up on them.
12. Do not show favouritism, or encourage cliques, or rely on spies.
13. Provide continuous coaching and instruction for staff who need to improve their contribution or skills.
14. Be prepared to discipline staff whose behaviour falls below the standards agreed. Be seen to be fair, informed and concerned.
15. Never reprimand staff in the presence of others (unless a formal disciplinary interview when staff request representation).
16. Be an active source of information; do not let staff have to ask for information or rely on rumours. Hold regular meetings, provide notices and memos.
17. Be prepared to lend a hand with difficult tasks, or when short-staffed. Avoid taking over or interfering.

These general guidelines for responsible management can be applied by both 'direc-

Directive management	Consultative management
1 Set clear objectives, targets and standards for a unit.	1 Reach agreement on objectives, targets and standards for a unit.
2 Set clear priorities for each job.	2 Agree clear priorities for each job.
3 Hold regular review sessions with individuals and teams to provide them with feedback.	3 Hold regular review sessions with individuals and teams for mutual discussion and feedback.
4 Introduce new approaches aimed at improving unit effectiveness.	4 Encourage staff to make suggestions for improvement. Take suggestions seriously. Give constructive response.
5 Encourage staff to take training useful to the unit.	5 Encourage staff to be self-developing.
6 Hold regular briefing meetings.	6 Hold regular meetings which are participative in style.
7 Maintain some distance from staff. Retain some formality.	7 Do not accentuate differences in rank, qualifications, experience, age or status. Aim for informality.
8 Be decisive and authoritative.	8 Be authoritative but considerate.
9 Require staff to report results regularly. Define individual responsibility.	9 Encourage staff to help each other. Encourage flexibility and collective responsibility.
10 Inform staff when changes are necessary for improved efficiency. Plan changes first.	10 Consult staff in a genuine way whenever changes or problems arise. Plan only after consultation.

Fig. 14.1 Some characteristics of extremes of management styles.

tive' and 'consultative' managers. In considering a particular situation, a nurse manager may wish to modify her style, either to become more directive or more consultative. Some of the main characteristics that need to be developed are shown in Figure 14.1.

MANAGERS AND POWER

To be successful in influencing the behaviour of other people in work in a positive way requires not only the choice of an appropriate leadership style, but also the possession of some source of power to reinforce this. This is necessary in the direct relationship between manager and line subordinates, but is even more essential in the relationships with fellow medical and nursing professionals or with staff in more senior posts.

Today, both in the NHS and independent hospitals there is considerable pressure on ward sisters to exercise skills in 'peer management' and 'boss management' as well as to develop power to be an effective leader of a staff team.

Sources of power

In a relatively straightforward line relation-

ship, the more senior post has formal authority to instruct more junior staff within the official rules and procedures and, when necessary, to apply disciplinary sanctions. Where junior staff accept the legitimacy and reasonableness of instructions, then authority is supported by practical power. This can be termed 'positional power'.

Most work relationships are not as simple as this. Junior staff often have power to resist senior directives or to influence their behaviour. Staff at the same official level in a hierarchy but in different departments will, in theory, have no authority over each other but, in practice, one may have power to influence the other.

In a hospital the highest authority figure should be the district general manager, but in practice more power might be held by a consultant or registrar, COHSE shop steward or even the head porter.

One source of such practical power is derived from being recognised as more knowledgeable and experienced than others — this is 'expert power'. Such personal credibility means others will seek your advice or defer to your suggestions. Staff working in specialist and advisory roles have to develop an expert power base.

One of the most difficult relationships for sisters/charge nurses is with younger, less experienced medics. In theory the doctor has greater expertise on medical treatment, but in reality he can benefit from the depth of experience and accumulated knowledge of certain patients and medical treatments possessed by senior nurses. Thus instead of waiting passively for the medical expert to direct the next stage of patient treatment, the nurse can suggest, using tact and subtlety, appropriate action to be approved by the doctor. Thus she influences his behaviour by using unofficial, yet significant, expert power.

There will be similar circumstances for a sister nominally reporting to a senior nurse who does not have as much direct experience or training in the specialisation of the particular ward. It is essential to take the initiative in requesting resources, indicating problems and proposing developments.

Another source of power can come from having control over resources that are in short supply. Thus in the formal organisational structure, the head porter may appear to be at a lower level of authority than the director of nursing services but can exercise considerable influence on what actually happens in a hospital. The senior nurse responsible for the provision of 'bank nurses' to cover staff shortages will also have resource power, as will ward sisters if they discriminate in the amount of co-operation they exhibit towards different doctors.

Managers will experience the irony of occupying a post of authority over staff but then finding that the manager needs staff support and co-operation more than they need his. The most powerful groups in most organisations are at the top, if they control appointment of staff, allocation of investments and devise the overall structure; at the bottom of the hierarchy where they can control work practices, work quality and work output; and in specialist posts of strategic importance (computer staff, medical staff). The least powerful positions are those of middle and junior management. There must be an effort by middle managers to build up their expert and resource power bases if they are to exert an influence on the top and bottom stratas of the formal health care hierarchy.

TEAM BUILDING

It is likely that an analysis of most situations in health care will suggest a priority need for managers to create a unit where staff combine their efforts as an effective team. At the more senior levels of health care management, there has been an emphasis on this need to have co-operation and co-ordination between the various disciplines. Criticism has been directed at the NHS management in failing to form genuine collaborative work groups; instead sectional interests seem to prevail.

Nurse managers will be involved in several team working situations. They will be leaders of a permanent group of staff whose combined efforts are necessary for the successful working of a unit. Senior nurses are also members of other teams such as the nursing management team, specialist health care team and occasional project teams.

It is useful to give particular consideration to team leading and team building. A team is not just a collection of individuals thrown together in work. A team is a group of people united by shared values, objectives and a desire to complete specific work tasks. They are dependent on each other and help each other. They recognise that their combined efforts are likely to produce better results than they could achieve individually. Unless there is such commitment the use of the label 'team' will not in itself unify a collection of individuals.

The characteristics of an effective team can be summarised as:

1. Individuals allocate their priorities towards team goals.
2. Individuals consider the impact of their actions on the rest of the team.
3. Individuals consult with each other before significant decisions.

4. Individuals keep each other informed about activities, problems and achievements.
5. There is helpful competition and constructive conflict of ideas.
6. Conversations at team meetings are open and honest.
7. Conversations about work are the same inside and outside work.
8. Meetings are productive and stimulating.
9. New ideas abound.
10. Ideas are translated into effective action.
11. There is group ownership of ideas.
12. There is regular, open review of team effectiveness.

Such team spirit can arise spontaneously if there is mutual recognition of the need for collaboration. Nursing auxiliaries, in getting through the physically demanding tasks of caring for high dependence, long-stay patients, may help each other without any outside influence. Medical and technical staff help each other to solve problems that are beyond the grasp of any single expert.

Where there is a need to foster team spirit, attention should be given to a number of points:

1. Clarification by individuals of the collective aims and purposes
2. Recognition of the role each individual plays in the team effort
3. Recognition that team success depends on all members contributing
4. Encouragement of the view that all members share the responsibility for achieving team aims
5. Encouragement of direct and open communication between all staff
6. Encouragement of flexibility and mutual support between members
7. Encouragement of social interaction of all members during breaks, etc.
8. Provision of learning opportunities and experiences for all team members
9. Use of team slogans, names and culture to reinforce feelings of belonging
10. Publication and celebration of team achievements.

In considering ways to improve management team working, some research findings may be useful (Belbin, 1981). This suggests that teams should not have more than seven members and that each member plays a 'functional' role (particular expertise, representative of section, etc.) and a 'team' role, which is an additional contribution to the processes of team working. These team roles should not be allocated according to seniority but according to the needs of the group and the personal qualities of the individuals.

Eight distinct roles are identified:

chairman, shaper, plant, monitor/evaluator, company worker, team worker, resource investigator and completer.

Although practical nurse managers may doubt whether such an elaborate structure of roles could actually be allocated to an existing health care team, it is useful to consider the mechanisms of team working. It is unlikely that a group of individuals selected for various functional roles and professional expertise, and representing sectional and individualistic interests, will automatically form into a cohesive team. When setting up project teams, the size, composition and team roles should be discussed.

MANAGING RELATIONS WITH SENIORS

There are many books, research studies and training courses addressing the topics, 'How to be a good boss' or 'How to manage staff'; as yet much less attention has been directed to the equally important question, 'How to manage your boss and other senior figures'.

The reason for this omission is the underlying assumption of hierarchical organisation structures. Those appointed to the more senior positions are supposed to possess superior knowledge and wisdom to those in more junior posts. Therefore, seniors are expected to make decisions and to lead, whilst juniors are expected to provide information, carry out allocated work tasks and apply the decisions of their superiors. This is a simplification of the reality of how organisations work in practice. Many seniors have less technical knowledge than their staff, some have inferior decision-making skills and less direct experience of the work in their unit. In some parts of an organisation there will be junior staff pushing their bosses into decisions and action, rather than waiting loyally for instructions to be passed down.

Influencing more senior managers depends on the exercise of available expert and resource power in an appropriately skilful style.

The ideal working relationship is one based on openness and respect, where a 'subordinate' feels confident in expressing views, taking initiatives, making suggestions, and where decisions are based on reasoned discussion. In such a situation good bosses will produce good staff. It is frequently necessary for staff to adopt less open tactics in an effort to improve the effectiveness of more senior staff, rather than take the easy way out of simply criticising 'the boss' behind her back.

In seeking to influence, or even manipulate, it is useful to develop an understanding of your manager. Try to appreciate how she is treated by her seniors, what pressures she is under, what are the real limits of her authority, what are her motivations. You can work for managers who are very career oriented and mainly concerned about the image they project to higher managers, or you can work for managers who are concerned with producing results they feel are necessary, without much concern about who they upset in the process. Some managers are interested in details and like to be involved; others prefer not to know what is going on, provided there are no problems. Some bosses will stand up for staff when criticism is directed at failures and mistakes; others will happily blame them to save themselves from criticism. Some managers will give credit to their subordinates when meeting their own seniors; others will steal subordinates' ideas and claim them for their own. Thus the first principle of boss management, like staff management, is

to know the strengths and weaknesses of your boss. Then consider what she wants from you. One boss may be very knowledgeable, well established and confident, and thus be prepared to listen to argument or criticism. Another boss may be new, lacking knowledge and confidence, in need of help, encouragement and support from staff.

The basic choice for staff is whether to try to work with their seniors, or against them. Existing staff often feel resentful about the way their immediate supervisor has been appointed. This may lead them to become at best passive, if not definitely hostile. It is usually wiser to come to terms with the reality of a new appointment and seek to co-operate. In general it is possible to identify a number of qualities that most managers would like to find in junior managers and staff in their immediate span of control. They generally prefer staff who:

— Bring them solutions rather than just problems
— Are willing to take on work without having to be told
— Set high standards for themselves and their staff
— Know what is going on in their own section.
— Are well organised and efficient
— Are in touch with the feelings of their staff
— Are constructively critical, not destructive moaners
— Are consistent
— Are flexible
— Are trustworthy
— Are prepared to listen
— Support their bosses
— Above all else, produce results.

It is possible to use some of the principles of good staff management in trying to get the best out of your more senior management. Give them regular praise; keep them in the picture; involve them in some of your decision-making; give them a feeling that progress is being made; give them the good news as well as the bad.

From this base you will be able to exercise

influence to ensure that appropriate decisions are made, that you are involved, and that you get a fair share of the resources that are available. If you do your best to fill the part of ideal subordinate, but do not get a fair response from your boss, you may be forced to adopt more assertive tactics.

There is a distinction between being assertive in relations with others and being aggressive. An assertive individual is concerned with exercising her rights, making sure others take account of her needs as well as their own.

In the last decade there has been considerable interest in training and encouraging women, in particular, to increase their assertiveness. Within the NHS, since the Salmon restructure in 1974 there has been an increase in male appointments to senior posts, with this trend continuing after the introduction of the Griffith proposals. Thus it continues to be a priority for female nurses and nurse managers, in particular, to assert themselves.

If a positive approach to developing constructive relationships fails and reasonable assertiveness does not improve matters, a junior will have to resort to more aggression and self-protection from an exploitative or totally ineffective boss.

Such last resort strategies involve going over the head of the manager to an appropriately powerful, more senior and hopefully more sympathetic manager, in order to put forward problems and recommend solutions.

It is possible in extreme cases to exercise one's right under the Grievance Procedures or professional codes of conduct after seeking appropriate advice from officers in a trade union.

Protective devices involve keeping scrupulous records of your own actions, putting out memos and reports, either requesting decisions or confirming instructions that have been given verbally, so that you maintain evidence of the manager's malpractice and your own good efforts. Clearly, such negative approaches to managing indicate a breakdown in relationships.

REFERENCES

Adair J 1983 Effective leadership, Pan Books, London
Barnard L, Walsh M 1981 Leadership:the key to professionalisation of nursing. McGraw Hill, Maidenhead
Belbin M 1981 Management teams. Heinemann, London
Blake R, Mouton J 1978 The new management grid. Gulf Publishing, New York
Blake R, Mouton J, Tapper M 1981 Grid approaches for managerial leadership in nursing. C V Mosby, St Louis
Clark M 1978 Getting through the work (In: Dingwell R, McIntosh J(eds)Readings in the sociology of nursing. Churchill Livingstone, Edinburgh
Epstein C 1982 The nurse leader, Reston Publishing Inc, Reston, Virginia
Feilder F 1967 A theory of effective leadership, McGraw-Hill, Maidenhead
Hersey P, Blanchard K 1977 Management of organisational behaviour. Prentice Hall, New Jersey
Lickert R 1961 New patterns of management. McGraw-Hill, Maidenhead
Tannembaum R, Schmidt W 1958 How to choose a leadership pattern. Harvard Business Review

15
Managing the introduction of changes

MANAGING CHANGE

Health care workers, in common with staff everywhere, are increasingly affected by change. Developments in medical technology, new practices in patient care, administrative reorganisation, different patterns of staffing, alterations in training programmes, are a few of the pressures that bring change upon nurses and their managers. These can be regarded as the 'driving forces'. There is a similar array of 'resisting forces' at work to counteract the drive for changes. Representatives of broad 'community' interests, representatives of employee interests and representatives of government may push in different directions, thus modifying or halting the processes of change. Internal representatives of different sections and different professional groups will also be part of the resistance. Every move towards modification of the status quo is welcomed by some as an opportunity but perceived as a threat by others.

Managers have a dual role in the processes of change. In some circumstances they are in the driving seat. They bring their professional and personal influences to encourage more senior nurses, health administrators, auxiliary managers, medical staff and patients, as well as their direct nursing subordinates, to support their new developments.

At other times they seek to modify or resist changes advocated by others, either within the nursing hierarchy, or from other sources. Every nurse manager who is expected to be part of an official programme implementing changes, who seeks to be an informal agent of change at unit level or tries to halt the introduction of undesirable change, will need an understanding of the strategies and skills of managing change.

THE IMPACT OF CHANGE

Advocates of the extended nursing role or the application of the 'nursing process' see benefits to patient care and the status of the nursing profession. Many practical nurses on the other hand are sceptical, regarding these changes as a source of extra work with little advantage either to themselves or their patients. Many doctors have had similarly critical reactions.

The main driving force for NHS changes should be a desire to improve the standard of patient care or to provide existing standards at lower costs. Thus the dispassionate analysis of any proposed change should start with two broad questions:

1. What are the likely benefits to the services of our hospital or community service from this change?
2. What are the likely threats to the services provided or the efficiency of our hospital or community service from this change?

If the benefits appear to offset threats the change would have some justification. Often the driving force is insufficient funds in the district/hospital budget to meet costs. In some circumstances the best it is possible to claim is that resultant changes, although bringing no positive benefit, do not actually threaten services.

In some circumstances, however, a general manager would suggest a benefit of cost saving without reduced services, whilst medical staff would make the opposite analysis. This was the case at the Maudsley Hospital (Sunday Times 1986) in S.W. London in May 1986 when changes, including closure

of an emergency unit and merging of a drug addiction unit with an alcoholics unit, were proposed by the district general manager but strongly resisted by staff.

A manager seeking to advance change of this magnitude has to anticipate such reactions and to realise that either the change is unrealistic, or to consider means of coping with the resisting factors.

A similar analysis should be made at unit level by a senior nurse as a preliminary to seeking change.

In one case a newly appointed nursing officer had taken over the responsibility for three wards in a special eye unit of a general hospital and found the sisters and staff nurse had been allocated to specific wards on a permanent basis. The nursing officer believed there were benefits in terms of patient care and efficient ward administration if staff became more flexible and interchanged. This had been the practice in her previous hospital.

Thus when there are potential organisational benefits, the next stage should be an evaluation of the likely impact on staff. Two broad questions need to be answered:

1. What are the likely benefits to staff in your hospital or community service from this specific change?
2. What are the likely threats to staff in your hospital unit or ward from this change?

Whether an individual perceives a proposed development as a threat or a potential benefit depends partly on the amount of information he has and how he relates it to his self-interests. Some apparent resistance to change can be caused by misunderstanding by management, as well as by staff.

The nursing officer wanting staff to be more flexible between wards may not fully understand the practical problems this could create in the same way that staff do not properly understand how it could be organised.

Effective communication does not necessarily reduce resistance to change. By fully understanding the possible benefits to patient services or hospital efficiency weighed against the likely impact on themselves, staff may still consider the change undesirable. The potential benefits/opportunities and threats to staff are summarised in Figure 15.1. Some results of change are likely to be interpreted as a threat by all staff — less pay, longer hours, reduced choice in time-off, etc., — while other aspects will be regarded by some staff as a benefit but by others as a threat — more responsibility, changed location, redundancy, extra training, etc. Thus in trying to anticipate the reaction of others it is necessary to appreciate their point of view: How will they

react, not how 'should' they react.

It will be valuable to consider some potential change in a part of the health service with which you are familiar and attempt this analysis. Here it is also necessary to assess whether individuals or representative bodies are likely to have an interest and whether they will react favourably or otherwise.

CONTROLLING CHANGE

The planned introduction of change can go

Factors in job satisfaction	Threats	Opportunity/benefits
Security	Loss of job	Redundancy pay/early retirement
Pay and allowances	Reduced earning through regrading, less overtime, etc.	Increased earning through upgrading, bonus, overtime, etc.
	Lose extra pay, expenses, allowances	More expenses, allowances
Job interest	Less variety	More variety (job enlargement)
	Less responsibility	More responsibility
	Less autonomy	Less close supervision
	More responsibility	Less responsibility
	New location	New location
Work effort	Harder manually	Less manual, more mechanical aids
	More paperwork	Less paperwork
	More stress	Less stress
	Longer hours	Shorter hours
	Fewer breaks	More breaks
Conditions	Less convenient hours	More convenient hours
	Less favourable 'off duty'	More favourable shifts
	Less choice on holidays	More holiday choice
	More health/safety hazards	More safe and healthy
Job challenge	Less skill/more skills	More skills needed (job enrichment)
	No training available	Extra training
Training compulsory	Better quality	
	Pressures to learn	Learning opportunities
Career prospects	Fewer senior posts	Promotional opportunities
	Less learning opportunities	Extra skills, qualifications
	Less movement	Transfers possible
Status	Downgraded	Upgraded
	Lose privileges	Gain privileges
	Reduce own 'empire'	Increase own 'empire'
	Less influential	Increase influence
Social	More isolated	Join good team
	Break up work team	Team recognition
	Move from friends	Maintain friends
		Meet new people

Fig. 15.1 Likely impact of change on staff.

through three main stages:

1. Preparation
2. Implementation
3. Consolidation and follow-up.

Preparing for change can involve a range of activities depending on the driving force. Some managers would undertake research and consultation, involving their staff, colleagues, seniors, and trade union representatives in project teams or discussion groups, with the intention of really understanding the practical issues and potential problems before final decisions are made. This approach might lead into some negotiation, either in an attempt to draw up an official agreement to implement change, or more informally to establish an understanding of how it will work.

Other managers, either from personal preference, or as they are more constrained by the circumstances, would elect for a more educational or persuasive approach. The aim is to 'soften up' those who may oppose the manager's wishes, using verbal and written presentation, probably incorporating some assurances on the main points of concern (no compulsory redundancy, training to be provided, trial period with review, possible upgrading, etc.).

Less open strategies involve attempts to manipulate or coerce others into acquiescence. These managers identify key opposing figures, then seek to persuade, buy off or dispose of them. They may use rumours or distort information. Finally, they make threats of closure, dismissal or career disadvantage to win over opponents.

The main factors to be considered when choosing a strategy for change will include: level of likely resistance; significance of change; amount of leeway available to manager; time available; power and authority of proposers and likely opposers of change; preferred management styles; work custom and practices; prevailing organisational culture; trade union recognition and presence; staff expectations; support from higher authority.

Although there are no universally correct ways of preparing for change, the best management approach would involve research and consultation. This is likely, not only to identify ways to make changes work out in practice, but also to gain maximum commitment from those affected. If this approach does not produce voluntary co-operation, the other options of persuasion and coercion remain available.

In some organisations, however, with very entrenched attitudes and work practices (these are likely in management circles as well as amongst junior staff), a manager may consider a more threatening approach as the only way to 'unfreeze' complacency. This is calculated to cause disruption and confrontation, but the manager would then 'soften up' other managers and staff to be prepared to co-operate in a more consultative exercise afterwards.

An effective preparation phase will allow managers time to plan and to obtain the necessary co-operation to implement changes properly. There are many examples where managers have tried to rush matters only to find unexpected difficulties and staff reacting in a 'we could have told you' manner. Using the techniques of project planning described in Chapter 3 should ensure the proper introduction of new procedures, new equipment, new treatments, etc. Successful implementation also depends on effective monitoring and control, so that initial difficulties are dealt with quickly and unanticipated events overcome.

Attention to getting things right in the first place will increase a manager's credibility with her staff, with her senior managers, with her colleagues and all others who are aware of the effort that has been made. Once a new system seems to be working it is important for management to keep any promises for training, improved facilities, upgrading, etc. that were made in the preparation stage.

It is also important to obtain information that shows the promised benefits in improved service or efficiency have been achieved.

Preparing for change — management strategies

1 Consultation and involvement by management with those with interest in the need to change to explore views and identify acceptable outcomes.

or

2 Education and communication by management to sell the benefits of change to those likely to be affected.

or

3 Negotiation and assurances by management to make a bargain to offset disadvantages of change.

or

4 Manipulation by management to undermine resistance and opposition.

or

5 Coercion and direct action by management to impose change.

Fig. 15.2 From an analysis of potential opportunities/threats to staff there are five distinct ways to introduce change. Health care managers may also feel a need to monitor the outcome of changes that they are forced to accept. This will enable them to refer back to health authorities and administrators with evidence that promised benefits did not happen and to enable them to suggest acceptable modifications or to put up more credible resistance to future inappropriate changes.

REFERENCES

Lancaster J, Lancaster W 1982 The Nurse as Change
  Agent C V Mosby, St Louis
Sunday Times Report 1986 May 11th

16
Managing human problems in work

MANAGING STRESS

All work in the caring professions can be difficult. Patient care, whether in hospital or in the community, involves emotional and physical strain from contact with people in distress, whilst working long hours with inadequate resources. As a result, although there are also immense satisfactions in medical work, everyone with substantial nursing experience will be accustomed to the problem of stress; for nurse managers these problems are likely to increase, however. There is an additional responsibility of helping staff cope as well as additional personal pressures from an extended role.

Stress can arise when any individual feels under pressure at work (or in social/domestic life), although this is not an inevitable response. Intellectual, emotional, or physical strain is beneficial where the individual is able to develop the necessary attitudes and skills to cope effectively. It is only when we are unable to call on reserves of ability and energy that stress will be experienced. Thus any situation can be stimulating and enjoyable or stressful and threatening, depending on personality and experiences of the individual, although there are some generally acknowledged circumstances in work which tend to be stress-inducing.

The most obvious is simply an outcome of pressures created by having too much work but too little time and resources. This

139

becomes particularly acute when work is also of a standard beyond an employee's ability, or where exact deadlines and standards have to be met.

Ironically, stress can also be created in the opposite situation when not enough work is available to keep an employee busy, or where it is of a low quality with little intrinsic interest or purpose.

Other circumstances that contribute to stress are working in 'ambiguous' surroundings. This results when we are not clear on standards of work required; on what the future prospects are; when we have several bosses; or when we are at the focus of conflicting demands from senior staff. Ward sisters may feel anxious about the appropriate relationship with doctors, whether they are really managers, senior staff or colleagues, and about conflicting demands between nursing standards and resources available from health authorities.

Stress symptoms

Such pressures are widespread, both in business and in public service organisations, but, although not inevitably producing stress responses, many individuals will experience feelings of tension.

This may be expressed outwardly by more irritable behaviour than normal, or more impatient and aggressive behaviour. Alternative reactions can be difficulty in concentrating or thinking clearly, and a preference for focusing on short-term issues. Another variation on normal behaviour may be excessive concern with trivia or an anxiety to have everything correct.

There is often a tendency to reduce communication with others, especially where difficult relationships are a source of tension, while defensive behaviour becomes characteristic — the irony being that in difficult circumstances benefit can be obtained from talking to others and seeking advice. Unfortunately, this not only becomes less likely, but there is a greater tendency to take unilateral action, rather than seek co-operation and approval,

thus aggravating the situation and further increasing tensions.

Health risks can be increased for individuals working long term under stress. Job pressures can induce heavier smoking, drinking and over-eating as well as reducing the opportunity for exercise and time-off for family and leisure activities. Nurses should, by training and professional experience, be well equipped to detect such stress-induced changes in their own and other people's behaviour.

The practical problem in helping others over stress is that alterations in 'normal' behaviour or life-style may be difficult to detect, or may not be caused by work. Similarly, in trying to overcome the problem ourselves we may not recognise, or be prepared to acknowledge, symptoms. Thus pressures continue to mount until there is a serious reaction in the form of breakdown or total withdrawal by the individual.

This general tendency for stress to be part of work experience is applicable to managers, but such jobs have additional stress-inducing elements. This is as true for nurse managers as it is for hard-pressed executives in business. In direct nursing, although the work can be hard, there is an easily identified purpose and tangible reward in caring for patients. Practical and well-recognised professional skills have to be used. On the other hand, senior nurses often find their work is somewhat ambiguous, dealing with paper more than with people, sometimes lonely, and the focus of the conflict between needs of nursing staff and the demands of health authority administration. There are several common features of management life that can be the source of unpleasant pressures. These include:

— Having to make decisions affecting lives and careers of staff who you know well
— Feeling unable to influence senior managers' decisions
— Feeling a lack of communication and information from seniors, colleagues or staff
— Having to go along with or implement decisions you do not agree with
— Feeling you have too little authority but too much responsibility

— Feeling you have too heavy a work-load
— Being unclear about the scope and responsibility of your job
— Feeling that you are not liked by your staff or your boss.

This may seem a rather gloomy picture of work in general and management work in particular. It is likely that pursuing a career in large organisations means that stress has to be accepted as an occupational hazard; thus one of the skills of professional management is being able to develop strategies for helping oneself and others cope with it.

Increased irritability
Excessive concern with trivial issues
Poor decision-making — procrastination or stereotypical responses
Unreasonably sensitive to rumour
Reduced tolerance of ambiguous situations
Excessive complaints about the organisation
Highly critical of the work of others
Dissatisfaction with own job
Sense of futility
Difficulties in talking constructively with others
Feeling of tension and anxiety
Increased absenteeism
Tendency to overeat
Increased drinking or smoking

Fig. 16.1 Stress symptoms.

Coping with stress

A first stage can be to offer help, or seek help, through supportive conversation. There is considerable cathartic benefit in simply talking to someone sympathetic. A conversation between people who work together can also result in practical suggestions for removing some of the causes of stress (see next section on counselling).

If the problem is recognised as an excessive work-load, this might be eased by better delegation (upwards as well as down), by providing more staff, easing deadlines, revising priorities or using technical aids to ease pressure.

If the problems are the result of ambiguity of role and authority, representation to more senior staff might lead to some resolution. If the situation seems to be caused by lack of work, or work which is insufficiently demanding of an individual, there may be scope for job enrichment or for the job holder to try to expand the boundaries of the job. Such changes in the circumstances of a job can be carried out after discussion with those with the authority to make such changes. Alternatively, an individual, recognising the causes of his own problems, may make unilateral modification.

Another way of dealing with stress is to develop strategies for reducing the bad effects of pressure. Some practical steps which can be useful for managers to adopt include:

— Revising priorities in work to accept lower standards in some tasks or have less concern over some responsibilities
— Increasing self-discipline in not taking work home or worrying about work
— Improved planning of work and time management (see Chs 5 and 7)
— Taking full holiday and time-off entitlement
— Setting aside 'protection zones' at work, places to go, people to visit which are away from pressures
— Establishing friendships and supportive relationships in work
— Taking time out from a job to attend courses or visit other units
— Taking more regular exercise and pursuing outside interests
— Practising relaxation, yoga and meditation techniques in work when stress arises
— Taking more care of yourself, being positive in protecting yourself.

COUNSELLING

All people experience times of crisis in their lives. These may result from single traumatic events or may be perpetuated by more long-standing stress, frustration, anxiety, dissatisfaction and depression. Whether the cause is outside work, inside work or a combination, it is appropriate that we find someone to talk to.

Nurse managers will find it necessary, from time to time, to act as counsellor to staff, to colleagues and even more senior staff. This should be a natural role for members of a caring profession. It is useful, however, to consider what is involved in counselling, and whether a nurse manager can really be a counsellor to subordinate staff.

Often the cause of an individual's dissatis-fied feelings will be some aspect of work. In recognition of this, health authorities gave all staff the right to bring to the attention of management as a last resort the circumstances of a grievance by reference to an official griev-ance procedure. It is better practice for first-line managers to be sufficiently in touch with staff so that they discuss dissatisfactions before staff are forced to exercise this right.

First-line managers will also face the problem of dealing with staff whose standard of work or conduct has become unsatisfac-tory, but not sufficiently so to warrant disci-plinary action. In addition to such 'normal counselling', some managers encounter indi-viduals with more desperate problems leading them to the edge of a breakdown. Some managers also have staff members with personality inadequacies. In such circum-stances more profound 'crisis counselling' or some form of psychiatric help may be required.

Work in health care is stressful, but there should be available to ward sisters and senior staff access to suitably trained staff who are able to advise over such difficult staff problems.

This will not remove the need for line managers to be adept in counselling staff or in responding to staff grievances.

The basic aim in counselling is for the coun-sellor to be able to see a problem through the eyes of the person who is experiencing the problem. From this understanding of 'the facts' and feelings that lie behind the indi-vidual's sense of frustration, the counsellor should try to help the individual identify ways forward that may resolve the situation.

By listening to an employee a manager may hope that the complaint will be resolved by this process itself — talking through a problem often makes it disappear: if this is not the case then decisions on suitable action will be taken. Ideally, counselling is a slow process and is contrary to the normal pace of a supervisor's job. There are advantages to slowing down the rate of decision-taking in matters concerning relationships. Broadly there are seven stages in a counselling discussion. These can be summarised as:

1. Seeking understanding
2. Checking understanding
3. Seeking solutions from the individual
4. Testing solutions for practical difficulties
5. Summarising
6. Agreeing action
7. Follow-up

Expressed like this the counselling approach seems easy, and for some people it is. For many managers it is unnatural and difficult, as they are required to encourage someone else to talk, to listen carefully to what is said and to try to remove the problem of authority from the conversation. This is a change from a superior/subordinate relationship to a coun-sellor/client relationship.

It should be easy to understand someone's problem when he takes the initiative by talking with his boss, and where he is reason-ably articulate about his complaint. Unfortu-nately, many staff will be unable to describe their difficulties or grievances in a simple and coherent form, while others will be reluctant to approach management directly.

When a person has taken the step of asking to see his manager, care should be taken to ensure that the circumstances are suitable for counselling. Can you give the matter your full attention? Is the place quiet and free from interruption?

It will be important at the outset of the conversation to check that the correct procedures are being followed. In some cases a member of staff may be upset about treat-ment he has received from his immediate superior and thus be anxious to by-pass the procedure, taking the problem to a more senior manager or to someone in personnel. This creates a delicate situation · as the manager will not want to put off a disgruntled employee but equally should not undermine another manager. The choice of strategy is between seeking a brief understanding of the issue and then involving the supervisor, or referring the employee to the correct procedure.

Another practical problem may arise if a trade union representative brings a grievance direct to management when the first stage of procedure should normally be a meeting between the employee and his first line supervisor.

Assuming that there are no procedural problems and the time and place are right, the manager's task is to get the employee to talk through the problem.

Initially, the conversation may be difficult as the individual could be upset or hesitant, or suspicious. Thus the manager has to show sympathy, help the individual to feel at ease and encourage her to open up. He can do this by asking simple 'open' questions — 'Tell me what's up', 'Describe in your own words what the problem is'. At this stage some prompting may be helpful so that the individual is encouraged to give more information. 'That's interesting — go on.' 'Tell me more about it.' Where someone is being reticent there is a temptation to put words into his mouth and ask 'closed' questions — 'So you feel badly done by over this?', 'You did understand what was involved of course', 'So now you want to reverse the decision?' This temptation should be avoided.

Once somebody is talking reasonably freely it is advisable to probe for a deeper understanding of what he is saying. Asking people what they mean by the words they use and what lies behind their opinions *in a helpful way* is the basis of the art of probing — 'What do you mean when you say that the arrangements were unfair?', 'How long have you felt like this?', 'Did you say anything at the time?'

Again this sounds simple and again for some of us it is. There are problems in

adopting this style of conversation between manager and subordinate. The manager will often feel a need to defend her actions or the hospital policy. If a nurse says, 'This department is a dump', when counselling, a Sister should ask for reasons. But she may feel an urge to argue the point and to describe the difficulties she has in trying to run the department.

There is a problem for a manager listening to a subordinate when she feels there is a flaw in the subordinate's reasoning or understanding. The temptation may be to point out aggressively where the other person is wrong.

Putting people down and scoring points at their expense are common features of encounters at work. Such approaches are inconsistent with a counselling relationship. It is possible, instead, to show someone his inconsistencies, or lack of information in a sensitive way, avoiding his resentment.

In any conversation, listening properly requires effort on our part. It is natural to listen and think at the same time. What one person says will stimulate thought in others, either to be used in reply or to distract them from what else is being said. In counselling the sequence should be: A asks B for his views, listens carefully and asks B to expand and explain, whilst showing empathy to B.

Another difficulty in manager/staff counselling is that the past experience of the manager may create prejudice — 'They're always moaning in this place', 'She's useless anyway' — which causes her to close her ears and her mind.

Being aware of these pitfalls should help the nurse manager — counsellor and prevent conversations degenerating into arguments or fatherly pep talks.

When a manager has got an individual to talk openly and to elaborate so that the picture is reasonably clear, it is good policy to check that she really has got it right by going over the information gathered. 'Let's see if I've got it right — last week you were expecting to be offered overtime but . . . ' The process of telling the story back is likely to lead the manager to ask more questions and the employee to add more detail until the picture is clear.

If a manager can appreciate what has been bothering an individual, a solution to the problem may emerge in that the individual may have been misinformed and simple clarification is all that is needed. Alternatively, the manager may become aware that the problem or grievance is well founded and that a change is required to rectify it.

In counselling it is most appropriate to see if the individual has a view on what should be done about his problem; the manager will then have to assess the practical implications of the employee's request — 'Will it upset other staff?', 'Is it in line with policy?', 'Will it cause problems in the future?' Ideally, the manager should resist telling an employee why his requests are impractical (assuming that they are). Instead, she should seek to explore the extent to which the other person understands these practical problems. 'How do you think other staff will react if we grant you the extra holiday?', 'How much do you think that will cost?', 'What will happen next year?'.

There are several advantages in asking a person for ideas to solve his own problem. In some cases he may not want any further action. Simply bringing the matter to the attention of management is enough. If practical suggestions are forthcoming and they are acceptable, it is more satisfying to have put these forward than having the same solution suggested by someone else. There is also the pitfall in offering the obvious answer to someone else's problem of getting a negative response — 'I couldn't do that'. 'It won't work'.

Difficulty may be encountered when the member of staff requests, or demands, action that the manager cannot approve or authorise. The choice of action is between ending the conversation so that the parties involved can think over the problem and meet again; summarising the failure to reach agreement and informing the individual of his rights under the grievance procedure; or trying to find an alternative solution.

At the end of a meeting it is good discipline for the manager to sum up what has been discussed and, most importantly, what action has been agreed. It is also good management discipline to make notes about the conversation, actions agreed and to make arrangements for any follow-up necessary. This is most important where a conversation has ended on a positive note with the manager promising to do something. Failure to carry out the promise in practice will create more grievances and bad feeling.

An employee who complains may be considered an inconvenience in some circumstances, but there is a great advantage in having something in the open as it is then likely to be resolved. It is more unsatisfactory to have murmurings of discontent in a department and clearly something a manager needs to counteract. Sisters should be aware of moods and morale, by regular informal contact and adopting a reasonable counselling approach — listening and understanding — in everyday conversations.

It would be naive to suggest that all troublesome and disgruntled staff will respond to such an approach and have their difficulties instantly resolved. Many managers report that once the ice has been broken the outcome is more gratifying than they imagined.

The principles of the counselling approach should form a sound base for managers wishing to develop satisfactory relationships with staff; incidentally it will do them no harm in dealing with their management colleagues.

BEHAVIOUR MODIFICATION

The aim of counselling is to help an individual identify the source of problems and to find ways of either coping with, or preferably overcoming, them. This should lead to the restoration of normal behaviour and a return to satisfactory work performance, but counselling does not always produce these desired results.

An alternative approach with staff who tend towards some undesirable behaviour in work is to try direct action — trying to treat the symptoms without seeking a preliminary understanding of the causes. This is based on a simplified version of 'behaviour modification' processes used in teaching and therapy.

The application by management requires a manager first to be able to pinpoint the unsatisfactory behaviour that she wishes to change in a subordinate or behaviour which she wishes to encourage. This desired behaviour should be job related and expressed in specific tangible terms which could be quantified. If several aspects of job behaviour are of concern, the most important should be selected. It is then suggested that two forces concerning the particular behaviour pattern should be considered. These are:

1. The events or cues that precede the undesirable/desirable behaviour — the triggers
2. The possible benefits the individual feels result from his behaviour — the rewards or pay off.

In theory a change in the trigger or the potential pay off which seems to be associated with the selected behaviour might produce the desired modification.

REFERENCES

Bailey R 1985 Coping with stress in caring. Blackwell Scientific Publications, Oxford
Claus K, Bailey J 1980 Living with stress and promoting well-being. C V Mosby, St Louis
Gleed E 1982 The supportive counselling role for ward sisters. In:Hazel, Allen (eds) The ward sister. Bailliere Tindall, London
Handy C 1976 Understanding organisations, Penguin, London
Herman Becoming assertive:a guide for nurses. D Van Nostrand, Wokingham
Mercer G 1979 The employment of nurses. Croom Helm, London
Stewart W 1983 Counselling in nursing, Harper and Row, London
Stubbs D 1985 How to use assertiveness at work. Gower, Aldershot

17
Managing conflict

CONFLICT IN WORK

In talking to managers and supervisors from many different organisations about the nature of their work, it is easy to reach the conclusion that in many cases managing is concerned mainly with trying to sort out differences with other people and between other people. The management of conflict is a fundamental, but often unrecognised, skill, for managers in all organisations.

It would be nice to believe that health care was different. All staff might be expected to work in harmony towards the common aim of meeting patient and community health needs. Such a belief is unrealistic. Managing in a hospital as much as managing in a factory is about resolving differences so that the purposes of the organisation can be achieved.

There are circumstances where individuals are pursuing different aims and are therefore in direct competition. This will be an extreme form of conflict. There are other circumstances where members of a team disagree on the best means to achieve their objective. This is also a form of conflict. Although being a participant in these situations can be uncomfortable (or possibly stimulating), such conflicts are not only inevitable but are an essential feature of freedom and change.

The list of potential conflicts waiting to confront nurse managers is endless. There is competition with other managers and representatives over the allocation of scarce resources. Some doctors make demands of ward staff which cannot be met without creating conflict with other doctors. Senior nurses may have to act as conciliators where members of staff disagree on application of policies, or have so-called 'personality clashes'. Sisters can become involved in disagreements between patients, with relatives and with ancillary staff.

It is easy to become aware of the destructive aspect of conflict:

— Time and energy expended over what seem to be trivial issues.
— 'Winning' a contest over someone else means that he 'loses', thus creating further animosity and reduced co-operation.
— Involvement in fierce hostility or competition can generate anxiety and poor decision-making.

There are positive aspects of conflict which should counterbalance the drawbacks:

— Conflict can create new ideas and bring improvement in working practices, standards and relationships.
— Managers and staff are forced to be more critical of themselves, their standards and the services they provide.
— Where others are prepared to oppose you, you are forced to consider their interests and ideas, leading to greater harmony in future.
— Conflict and competition create energy, stimulation and adrenalin.

Nurse managers should not be afraid of conflict, but should be committed to use it for constructive ends, whether as protagonists in disagreement or in the role of conciliator, seeking to resolve differences between others.

Symptoms and causes of conflict

Clearly two people in a heated argument could be a clear indication of conflict between them. Two managers sitting at a committee table presenting logical arguments which are intended to discredit the other are also expressing negative conflict.

These are open indications of difference but there are more subtle and hidden forms of destructive conflict in organisations:

— Hostility expressed by one group or individual towards another but not in their hearing — 'Our sister has got no interest in helping learners . . .', 'That unit manager is only interested in saving money . . .'
— Poor communication by deliberately keeping information from others or making decisions without consultation.
— Contact between staff deteriorates from formality to argument, and issues seem to become polarised.
— No goodwill, flexibility or co-operation. To get things done becomes more and more difficult.
— Many 'failures to agree' are passed up to higher authority for resolution.
— Problem situations are left untackled as individuals recognise the likelihood of unpleasant encounters if they take an initiative.
— Lots of sections consider themselves as 'us' and the rest as 'them'.

The basic cause of conflict is not personality differences or awkward individuals, but rather the result of different priorities between roles and departments, as well as different perspectives on means of achieving priorities. There will often be conflict between what an individual needs from work and what is required of the individual by an organisation. Trying to apply fair and flexible rota systems for part-time nursing auxiliaries can be difficult if this involves married women who also have demands of a home and family to consider. There will be other personal differences when individuals are competing for limited promotion or training opportunities.

HANDLING CONFLICT

If there are symptoms of underlying conflict, the managers with ultimate responsibility for running a smooth and efficient health service have a fundamental option. Either they take action, confront the problems and seek to resolve the conflicts, or they ignore the main issues, being content to treat symptoms when they become too extreme.

The temptation to ignore conflict in the hope that things will get better or from a belief that nothing constructive can be achieved, is understandable but is not really 'managing'. Thus we shall assume that a manager wishes to face up to problems.

We shall discuss two aspects of conflict management which are relevant to nurse managers — firstly as protagonists, either in interdepartmental conflict or within their units, and secondly as conciliators over internal unit differences.

Protagonist

As a manager trying to do the best for your unit there will be times when you seem to be drawn into competition with other managers and senior staff. At this point it is necessary to consider what strategies are available and which are likely to be adopted by others.

There are three common means by which managers try to resolve direct conflict. These can be called 'underhand' approaches, 'fair but tough' approaches and 'we can all win' approaches.

Underhand approaches

In most organisations there are underhand and unscrupulous dealings aimed at defeating those who are causing difficulties. These tactics may be used by manager against manager, by section head against members of staff or by staff against their management. The aim is destruction, or at least severe damage, to other people's position or influence. This is the destructive game of organisational politics. To play requires a ruthless determination and an accurate appreciation of power.

As a manager wanting a crucial decision to go in your favour, first identify who has the power to award this 'prize'. Consider how to

form a favourable alliance with him, by doing a favour or making a trade, lobbying with the strong points of your case and descriptions of the value of your unit. Make a better-prepared, better-researched and better-reasoned report than your opponents.

Underhand tactics are often directed at undermining the credibility of others, whether manager or staff. Such practices clearly signal a breakdown in human relationships and good faith, whilst putting self-preservation and expediency as the main justification for action. Upheavals in the ranks of senior management, appointment to top posts, the award of contracts, early retirements and resignations are sometimes preceded by such political activities. The health service is as much a scene of underhand conflict resolution as the seemingly more ruthless world of business.

Describing such management tactics is not to justify them but rather to acknowledge the reality of some aspects of organisational life. It also suggests that managers need to be alert to the politics of their own organisation and be prepared to counteract efforts made at backstabbing them.

To protect yourself it is useful to form alliances, to stick to procedures, to put on record your actions, to present a logical case on your own behalf and to be aware of your rights.

Fortunately, there are great risks in playing dirty as a manager. If you win you make enemies and need to be continually alert for counter-attacks from them or their allies. Then you might win the battle but lose the war — or you might simply lose the first skirmish and be totally discredited.

The fair but tough approach

This second form of competition is much safer and more constructive, although it is still based on the concept of one person trying to win so that others lose. The differences are that both parties openly acknowledge the competition, there are rules and a judge to decide the winner.

A unit manager's meeting can be the forum

for such open conflict. A senior nurse can be asked to present her arguments on a particular issue. The medical officer will then put forward his arguments. The meeting may continue in uncompromising attacks and counter-attacks until one side admits defeat, or the general manager awards the laurels to one protagonist.

If all parties accept this as game playing, to be carried out in order to make the best decision in the interests of the hospital, this may still lead to constructive conclusions and good relationships after the meeting. Unfortunately, some personalities get locked into the game by a desire to win, thus resorting to underhand tactics or seeking to overturn decisions by actions outside the meeting. Managers who seek to resolve differences by these rigorous confrontations run the risk of adversely affecting relationships which could lead to future destructive competition.

The we can all win approach

The preferred strategy in competition is to find ways in which all parties can feel satisfied with the result. This is particularly important where people have to collaborate to provide an effective service.

There are a number of ways in which it is possible to turn destructive aspects of direct conflict into constructive confrontation. None of these is difficult as long as at least one protagonist is aware of the nature of constructive difference. This rests on the distinction between arguing and discussing. If I argue with you my aim is to win by emphasising the logic of my views, by pointing out flaws in your reasoning and discrepancies in your data, supported by distortion, exaggeration and ridicule if necessary. The manner of an argument might change so that it is more persuasive and soft selling, but the essence remains that I am fixed in my assertions and it is likely that my rigidity will polarise your views. Deadlock will arise, or one of us will withdraw from the situation.

Discussion on the other hand starts from the premise that I at least will listen to your point of view. I will ask questions to understand your problems, your assumptions, your aims. In this I will try to find common ground, points of agreement and possible points of compromise. I will explain my position and expect you to listen and consider it. Discussion occurs between people with open minds and a willingness to co-operate. Argument happens between closed minds, each determined to beat the other.

In such constructive approaches to conflict there is still a need for managers to be rigorous and precise, at the same time being willing to consider other points of view. There is no creativity in seeking solutions to problems, unless the problems are really confronted.

Two constructive conclusions of discussion and consultation are either a mutual recognition of common interest and common needs, thus leading to a mutually acceptable solution, or an open recognition of difference but a willingness to compromise through negotiation. The conclusion of negotiation is a bargain that is a binding agreement or contract. I promise to accept your ruling but you promise to obtain extra staff for me. You are prepared to work the rota system but I accept you can change shifts with others if they are willing.

(A section on the techniques involved in management negotiations is included in Chapter 11.)

Even with the most constructive attitude between protagonists there will be situations which cannot be resolved. Agreement can still be made, however, to refer the matter to the next level of management or, in the case of interdepartmental disagreement, to the nearest level of general management.

Intermediaries

A manager of nursing staff is likely to be required to sort out some disagreements and clashes between staff. In such situations again there is a choice between whether to confront the issue or to ignore it in the hope that staff will sort it out themselves. Clearly, a responsible manager will wish to take some initiative to prevent conflict undermining the effectiveness of a unit.

Again, there is a choice. An undercover approach can be chosen in which a manager tries to improve matters by indirect action. Changing rota systems to keep people apart, trying to persuade one party to change behaviour, trying to catch them breaking rules so that disciplinary action can be taken, asking other staff to 'have a word', are likely tactics.

The alternative is to bring the staff who are in dispute together at a meeting for an open attempt at conciliation. In the role of intermediary the aim of a manager should be to encourage constructive behaviour. This can be achieved by:

— Asking one party to explain their point of view
— Preventing the other interrupting or arguing at this point
— Questioning the party to seek further clarification and justification of their actions and opinions
— Asking the other party to explain, questioning them and preventing the others from arguing or intervening
— Summarising the points of agreement, common interests and common ground between the parties, as well as the differences
— Putting forward possible solutions to test the reactions of each without commitment. It might be appropriate to meet each separately
— Trying to agree a mutually acceptable solution that is also of benefit to the unit
— If this fails, finally making an authoritative decision and making this into a binding agreement.

HANDLING DISCIPLINE

So far we have considered broad issues of conflict, but one aspect which affects all managers needs special consideration — this is the problem of staff discipline.

It is possible to define three main situations in which a nurse manager should be expected to take action as a result of undesirable behaviour by staff. One is when staff contravene, or ignore, some of the official procedures or codes of practice governing their work.

For example, in a hospital there are strict rules about the security and distribution of drugs and medicines which have to be followed exactly. Failure to obey regulations of this kind will involve employees and managers in serious disciplinary problems.

The second main source of disciplinary action arises from the problem of staff whose work falls below the acceptable standard. This can involve low quality treatments, shabby appearance, slow work, insufficient concern with patients' needs.

The most usual cause of disciplinary action, however, is where individuals fail to conform to general standards of good conduct. Cases of excessive lateness, unauthorised absence, unapproved breaks, misuse of property, may be quite widespread; while more serious incidents and dishonest behaviour are less common but may happen from time to time.

The fact that a nurse has apparently failed to follow official instructions or that her general approach is below standard, can be regarded as a management failure. Somewhere along the line of recruitment, selection, induction, job training, instruction or supervision, procedures are at fault. A professional response should be to investigate the circumstances and possible causes of each disciplinary situation. This can lead to informed judgement as to whether an individual case is the reflection of a more general weakness in personnel management systems, or really failure by one employee.

When a senior nurse has first-hand experience of a nurse's conduct, the next task is to seek reasons for its cause. When an incident has been reported by a third party it will be necessary to unravel several, possibly conflicting, versions of the same series of events. Preliminary investigation from records and other managers' information may be inconclusive. This poses a dilemma for a manager. Should she proceed and talk to individuals who are directly implicated, possibly accusing them falsely, or take no action in a situation which may deteriorate? In one such case a ward sister discovered that sleeping tablets were missing from a drugs cabinet and she suspected one nurse of taking them but had no proof. She had the choice of openly informing all staff of the problem, or keeping quiet in the hope of catching the culprit. Sister opted for the latter course and was subsequently accused of victimising a member of her staff who had a serious personal problem.

In talking to a member of staff as preliminary investigation into an apparent disciplinary breach it is important to do so in an open-minded way. Choose the most suitable time for the meeting which should be conducted in private. Decide who else should be involved and what notice should be given. If the approach is to be informal it is important not to ignore formal rights that staff have under a disciplinary procedure. If they wish to have a trade union representative, or colleague present, this should be arranged. Many experienced managers feel it is to their advantage as well to have a witness present, even at the informal stage of an interview.

There is a choice in how to structure such a meeting. A senior nurse can either present all the information she has and explain her reasons for being concerned, or she can ask the junior staff to give her point of view in response to a minimum amount of information. The advantages of starting with a full management statement is that it gives a nurse a clear picture of the background to the meeting. The disadvantages with this tactic are that staff may become defensive and angry at being, in their eyes, unfairly accused. The risk of confrontation is increased.

On balance, the advantages of seeking staff views without a manager committing herself suggest that this should be the preferred approach. If a nurse can be encouraged to talk openly it is likely that she will present information in a haphazard way. As listener it is necessary to check your understanding by occasional questions and summaries. In probing for details some standard points will be relevant:

— When did this happen?
— Who was there?
— Why did it happen?
— Was this the correct action?
— What should have happened?
— Who in authority was informed?
— What did they say or do?
— Has this happened before?
— How do you feel about this now?

By understanding a subordinate's view it is possible to compare this with your own understanding and identify discrepancies in a constructive manner. Avoid arguments and reprimands at this stage. The ideal conclusion at this point would be for a staff member to acknowledge her failings (assuming there are some), to describe the correct approach and agree for future improvements. This could be followed up with more training, closer supervision or clearer instructions. In practice, it is likely that issues will be more involved, probably being more grey than black and white with some faults on all sides. If the issue is not resolved at this informal stage, it may be wise to adjourn the meeting to seek more facts and consider the appropriate course of action. The basic management aims in more serious disciplinary problems are:

1. To rectify the undesirable behaviour of individuals concerned by counselling, coaching, instruction, disciplinary warnings or dismissal
2. To act fairly and be seen to act fairly towards all personnel involved
3. To follow good industrial relations practice by use of correct procedures and constructive behaviour
4. To give support to more junior management staff and to obtain support from more senior managers
5. To find ways of avoiding such problems arising in future.

In making a decision on whether to proceed beyond the informal stage with a disciplinary situation, it is helpful to take account of several considerations:

— How serious is the problem for unit efficiency, staff morale or unit reputation?
— What 'custom and practice' relates to the situation?
— What precedent might be set by management from action/non-action in the case?
— What is the record and quality of the particular employee?
— What are the likely responses of other staff to management action/non-action?
— What are the likely reactions from trade union representatives?
— What action is likely to gain support from higher management?

— What rules and procedures are applicable in the circumstances?

The formal disciplinary procedures are devised to have a series of regulated stages leading to the final sanction of dismissal. The most common procedure is one with four stages — verbal warning, first written warning, final written warning and then dismissal. There is usually an additional procedure for cases of 'serious misconduct' whereby dismissal may occur without the preliminary stages.

The principles involved in disciplinary interviews for the informal stages are applicable to the more formal disciplinary hearings. A manager must proceed with an open mind,

---

GUIDELINES ON HANDLING DISCIPLINARY PROBLEMS

MANAGEMENT AIMS

1. To investigate incidents or problems thoroughly before reaching decisions.
2. To treat individual in a fair and reasonable manner.
3. To correct individual behaviour where this is necessary.
4. To follow appropriate procedures.
5. To handle the situation in a way that is consistent with good industrial relations practice.
6. To prevent similar problems in the future.

MANAGEMENT APPROACHES

When an employee is observed or reported to have contravened rules, codes or standards that warrants some disciplinary action, a manager needs to investigate the circumstances.

1. Investigation

A manager needs reliable information which could be obtained from several different sources:
   Records (time-sheets, clock cards, production records, etc.)
   Official letters, contracts, notices, memos etc.
   Personal file of employee
This information may be enlarged by talking to people who have knowledge of the situation:
   Staff concerned
   Senior staff
   Patients
   Staff representatives
   Other staff
If the information obtained suggests further action is required a meeting with the employee will be arranged. Before this takes place the manager should consider:
   Who should be present? (employees, supervisors, staff reps., etc.)
   Where is a suitable private place?
   When is an appropriate time?
   What notice should be given?
   What preliminary information should be given?
   What information should be available at the meeting?
   Who should be standing by?

Fig. 17.1

---

2. Meetings

To achieve his aims a manager should consider the following points during a disciplinary meeting:

a. State the purpose at the beginning as 'investigation into complaint/problem'.
b. If a 'formal' hearing, advise the employee of his rights under the disciplinary procedure.
c. Briefly state reason for management concern in a calm and reasoned manner.
d. Invite employee to describe event and explain his views.
e. Use open style questions to encourage him to explain fully.
f. Question to enlarge understanding of his actions and views.
g. Establish:
    When and how long problem existed
    Where incident happened
    Who else was involved
    What was said by others
    Was any report made
    What was employee's understanding of official rules, correct conduct etc.
    What is employee's view of his behaviour now.
h. Summarise information and views given by employee.
i. Explain management view and give any conflicting information.
j. Attempt to resolve differences over interpretation of 'factual matter'.
k. Seek further information.
l. Consider an adjournment.
m. Summarise prior to adjournment.
n. Agree time for resumption.
o. Open meeting with summary of first part.
p. Ask employee if he has anything fresh to add.
q. Attempt to resolve any differences of interpretation of rules etc.
r. Summarise finally.
s. Explain decision to employee.
t. If no disciplinary action, agree any follow-up needed to help the employee — extra training, new instructions, more frequent reporting etc.
u. If disciplinary action, ensure employee and his representative understand this.
v. Advise employee on any rights of appeal.
w. End meeting by agreeing any additional follow-up — training, new instructions etc. — and on a positive note if possible.
x. Write up notes of meeting and decisions.
y. Inform superior, personnel, supervisor, other staff etc. as appropriate.

3. Style

The manager should remain calm throughout the meeting. It is advisable to start in a conciliatory manner with an open mind to avoid unnecessary confrontation.

4. Follow-up

At the end of a meeting a manager should consider:
    What caused the problem?
    Can anything be done to avoid this in future?
    What follow-up would help the situation?
    How well did management handle the situation?
    What could be improved on in management?

Fig. 17.1 (cont'd)

and seek to understand the staffs' view of events and any mitigating circumstances. Clear understanding of unit rules and instructions is essential, as is an understanding of the disciplinary codes and rights of representation. It is essential to make a comprehensive record of a case. Disciplinary procedures include a right of appeal. When this is exercised, managers must be able to demonstrate that disciplinary actions were based on full knowledge of the circumstances, the rules and the procedures involved. In the case of dismissal, employees have the right to take their case to an industrial tribunal where managers will need reliable and complete records of events (see Ch. 20).

At the end of a disciplinary matter, however it was finally resolved, it is sensible for managers to ponder about the basic causes. Employment policy should mean that an organisation employs competent staff who are willing to do a fair and responsible job. If a unit has frequent disciplinary clashes it may be a symptom of failure of this policy. Thus the effective management of discipline depends on management, not only acting fairly and in a business-like manner with particular problems, but also seeking to modify management practise and policy to prevent such problems arising in the first place.

REFERENCES

Handy C 1976 Understanding organisations. Penguin, London

Lewis D 1986 Essentials of employment law, Institute of Personnel Management, Wimbledon

Pyne R 1981 Professional discipline in nursing. Blackwell Scientific Publications, Oxford

Recruitment

Selection interviewing

Panel interviewing

18

Staff recruitment and selection

RECRUITMENT

Although only a few nurse managers are free to choose the staff they are required to manage, as most newly appointed managers take over an existing work team, it is still important for them to be skilled in the techniques used in the recruitment and selection of staff. Despite the obviousness of this point it is surprising how little time or serious thought is given to the task of filling vacant jobs.

When applying for a post in the National Health Service applicants are likely to be asked to fill in a simple application form and, if lucky, to attend a short interview. Here candidates are asked to respond to an apparently random selection of questions delivered in an intimidating manner by a panel of tense managers. These may allow applicants to present themselves in a favourable light, but are likely to leave them depressed and bewildered.

Yet out of this procedure important posts have to be filled. Mistakes are serious; not only do they hamper individual career progress, but jobs may be given to people lacking essential knowledge, skills or personal qualities. Clearly, staff recruitment is a vitally important task which should be handled competently.

To achieve professional competence in staff selection it is necessary to appreciate three main points: the aims and problems in selection, the procedures that can minimise the difficulties and the skills needed for effective selection interviewing.

Most nurse managers would state their aim in filling a vacant nursing post as: 'to find a competent individual who will fit in with the existing team'. There can be little argument about the need for competence but it is sometimes desirable to employ staff who will bring in new ideas and may stimulate a rather complacent team. Other aims in recruiting may be to provide career advancement opportunities for existing staff, and to conduct the whole exercise in a cost-effective and well-organised manner.

The usual starting point is clarification of the need for a particular appointment, and an outline of the purpose, responsibilities and tasks attached to it. This frequently involves the production of a written 'job description'. It is important that this is up to date and does accurately reflect the practical nature of the job. With a reasonably reliable description the next step is to decide what is required by an individual to carry out the function satisfactorily. This can involve the production of a 'person specification'. Using a list of headings which can be applied to all types of jobs can be helpful. There are several forms these can take, but most ask managers to consider the qualifications, skills, previous experience and personal qualities that are needed in a particular role. It may be wise to compile two

lists: one with absolutely essential features and the other with those that are desirable (see Figs. 18.1 and 18.2 for examples).

Within the NHS such 'person specifications' are not as widely produced as are official job descriptions. It is important for individual nurse managers or management teams to form considered views on what is required in each vacant post. There can be serious problems in this process. Beyond the basic professional qualifications the specification is a matter of personal opinion. Opinion is fallible and often based on untested assumptions about an ideal employee. Practical experience shows that a variety of personalities and work backgrounds can be adapted in the same work. There is no ideal profile for psychiatric nurses, ward orderlies or clinical nurse managers.

With agreement on the type of recruits required, the next stage of recruitment can be undertaken. This may involve some form of advertising. The choice of media for health service posts is relatively straight forward. There are well established professional journals for qualified staff and the local press and Job Centres for more junior appointments. When it is difficult to attract applicants it may be necesssary to use employment consultants, to run 'open days', to have post advertisements and to use local radio.

A good advertisement in the appropriate publication should instantly attract the casual

---

1. Physical make up
   Indicate requirements for health, eyesight, strength, hearing, stamina, appearance etc.
2. Attainments
   Indicate the level of general education, professional training and work experience.
3. Special Aptitudes
   Indicate any particular skills required — numeracy, handling money, creativity, sympathy with older people, word processing etc.
4. Intelligence
   Indicate any need for learning and problem-solving.
5. Interests
   Indicate any general interests or leisure activities that might be desirable
6. Disposition
   Indicate desirable or undesirable characteristics related to the job — working under pressure, working alone, teamwork, sensitivity, tolerance etc.
7. Special circumstances
   Indicate aspects of the job that make particular demands — shift work, mobility, unsocial hours etc.

Fig. 18.1 Person description. A seven-point checklist.

1. Educational qualifications and standards
   Indicate the general educational background required — CSE, degree etc.
2. Professional standards
   Indicate the professional and technical training and qualifications required.
3. Work experience
   Indicate the type of work experience required.
4. Special knowledge and skills
   Indicate particular work experiences, aptitudes, skills etc. required.
5. Personal qualities
   Indicate aspects of personality required or considered unsuitable.
   Indicate physical and health requirements.
6. Special circumstances
   Indicate special aspects of the job — shift working etc.

Fig. 18.2 Person description. A six-point checklist.

reader. There must be some indication of the attractions and rewards of a job, as well as the experience and qualifications required. The copy should be in concise but attractive style.

If all the preliminaries have been carefully followed it should result in a number of suitable enquiries for a vacancy. If there are more than a dozen it will be necessary to make a short list of those who are apparently most suitable. This initial selection should be handled with care. A beautifully typed and presented application form does not necessarily mean a beautiful and well-presented worker. Conversely, a poorly presented application does not mean an individual will not make a conscientious and caring member of a nursing team. Information provided in a written application should be compared against the key requirements of the person specification. Each applicant who seems to have the minimum needed under each heading should proceed to the next stage of screening. If this still results in too many to see personally, then other factors like preferred employment background, present location, employment stability etc. can be taken into account to draw up a manageable shortlist.

Throughout the public employment sector the formal interview is a central part of the staff selection process. Often this takes the form of a panel interview. This should not mean that this is the only method used to make appointments. The formal interview favours candidates who are able to anticipate questions and give 'right' answers, or those who are confident in giving spontaneous replies. Thus the interview can become a test of how good you are at being interviewed, rather than a means of revealing practical skills, professional knowledge, personal qualities and real motivation.

A comprehensive selection plan should put candidates into several situations to provide information relevant to their suitability for a particular post. It is common practice to invite prospective employees to see a workplace at first hand. During such a visit they will reveal some of their knowledge and experience, or lack of, concerning the type of work and facilities involved. In some occupations it is customary to bring 'samples of work' along to an interview. It is difficult for applicants to bring examples of clinical nursing or NHS administration, but it might be feasible for applicants for more senior posts to show examples of research studies, training schemes, staff development programmes and so on, which they have initiated.

It is becoming more common for organisations to use a variety of special tests for staff selection. The purpose is to provide 'objective' data about individuals which can be matched against the profiles in the 'person specification'. There are practical skills tests, tests of aptitude for specific types of work, tests of intelligence and inventories to reveal aspects of personality. Some tests are available to approved users and can be obtained from the National Foundation for Educational

Research (NFER), Nelson Publishing Company, Darville House, 2 Oxford Road East, Windsor, Berkshire.

It is possible to produce your own selection tests. If there is a need for written or numerical accuracy in a job, applicants can be given typical examples and asked to complete some. Where there is a need for sensitivity in dealing with other people, candidates can be placed in some group activity or individuals given a typical 'case' and asked to describe their approach to it. If there is a specific aspect of professional knowledge which is indispensable, then, rather than rely only on questions at an interview, it is possible to devise a written test paper to reveal knowledge of the subject.

In this DIY approach to selection testing it is important to make sure that tests will actually reveal the knowledge or aptitudes required. Can you do the test yourself? Can those already doing the job complete the test easily?

There are many critics of selection testing and a considerable amount of thought should be given to the problems as well as the advantages of tests. It is likely, even when tests are used, that there will still be heavy reliance on interviewing candidates.

SELECTION INTERVIEWING

If the preliminary stages of recruitment have been properly conducted it should mean that a manager will interview a few candidates, most of whom are capable of doing the vacant job, or can undertake training for it. The aim of interviewing is to make a fair assessment of each interviewee against each other and against the specifications in the 'person description'. This should lead to satisfactory appointment decisions. There can be two stages to an interviewing exercise. The first may consist of preliminary interviews conducted by personnel staff intended to screen out the more unsuitable applicants. This will be followed by final interviews involving the manager who is to 'employ' the selected appointee. Whatever type of interview there are three key characteristics of a satisfactory encounter:

1. Candidates should speak freely and openly about previous experiences, attitudes to work and any career aspirations.
2. Candidates should give direct information about professional or technical expertise related to the vacancy.
3. Candidates should obtain a clear understanding of the tasks involved in the job, the aims and responsibilities as well as the terms and conditions of employment.

Such two way communication should be easy to achieve. Yet we have all suffered at the hand of interviewers who ask a series of unrelated questions, who do not seem interested in our replies and only seem to have a hazy idea about the vacant job. These managers have not understood the basic principles of effective interviewing.

There are several barriers that an interviewer must overcome to develop a free flowing conversation. One is candidate stress. Most of us feel anxious about the uncertainty associated with going for an interview. This can make some candidates undersell themselves whilst others overcompensate for their nerves by overselling. A minority actually enjoy the interview game and present themselves in a favourable way. However this does not necessarily correlate with competence as a ward sister or nursing auxiliary. Tension is not restricted to the interviewee. The selectors are likely to feel ill at ease, forget to ask some important questions and fail to recall all that has been said to them. The whole process is subject to personal prejudice so that interviewers tend to feel an initial liking for a candidate and use the rest of the interview to confirm this impression. Alternatively, other interviewees will be written off after the first few minutes. Time is another serious difficulty. There is often insufficient time allowed for a thorough discussion with each candidate, and, with several interviews following in quick succession, interviewer fatigue may give some candidates unfair treatment.

```
┌─────────────────────────────────────────────────────────────────┐
│ Interview sheet                                                   │
│ Job title: _____        │
│ Department: _____        │
│ Candidate: _____   Interviewed by: │
│                                                                   │
│ Educational qualifications/Standards; _____         │
│ _____                │
│                                                    Checked Yes/No │
│ Professional standards: _____                 │
│ _____                │
│                                                    Checked Yes/No │
│ Work experience: _____                 │
│ Special knowledge and skills: _____                │
│ Personal qualities: _____                │
│ _____                │
│ Special circumstances: _____                 │
│ Summary/Recommendations: _____                  │
└─────────────────────────────────────────────────────────────────┘
```

Fig. 18.3 An interview report form.

In order to overcome these basic weaknesses in selection interviewing it is important to prepare properly for each one. This should take care of the obvious practical needs to book a suitable private room; to arrange suitable reception and waiting arrangements for each candidate; to be familiar with the content of application forms, letters, job descriptions, person descriptions and job conditions. Finally, it is useful to prepare an interview sheet so that notes can be made under the main headings of the person description.

A conventional selection interview can be broken into seven main stages:

1. The introduction
2. A broad 'biographical' review of a candidate
3. Specific questions on knowledge, skills and experience relevant to the vacancy.
4. Discussion of the job content, terms, conditions and organisational background
5. Questions from the candidate
6. Conclusion
7. Writing a summary of information gained from a candidate.

The opening minutes of the interview should help an applicant to feel more at ease and start to establish rapport with the interviewers. This can be achieved by exchanging a few pleasantries, smiling, referring to a candidate by name and giving a brief outline of the job. This should give candidates enough time to gather their thoughts. Some interviewers make the mistake of giving too much information about the job at this stage. It is wise to get an interviewee talking and to leave detail to later in the proceedings.

The introduction should lead naturally into asking applicants to answer straightforward questions about their career history to date. Here the main skills of interviewing are needed. This means asking appropriate questions in a short, 'open-ended' form that invite more than single word replies: 'What type of ward are you in at present?' 'What are the main tasks of your present post?' 'Why did you select that specialism after training?'

Once a candidate is talking freely the interviewer should listen quietly, then use a follow-up question to get a better understanding of what has been said or to fill in missing parts: 'In what way was this an unsatisfactory experience?' 'How many staff were in the team?' 'What did you do about accommodation?' If a candidate is shy in the early replies, encouragement may be needed by giving prompting remarks such as 'Go on', 'That's interesting' etc.; or to resort to more specific, but still open questions. There is a danger that an interviewer starts to use 'closed' questions which can be answered with a word or two.

'You did your training at the Royal?' 'You are still in the geriatric ward?' A shy interviewee will be monosyllabic in response, making the interviewer more uncomfortable. Closed questions should be used to establish basic facts. 'You will complete your training next month? 'Will you need accommodation if you leave?' If an expansive answer is required this may need a supplementary open question: 'Tell me about your training.' 'What arrangement can be made?' A good interview should develop into a natural conversation. In this way it is possible to gain a general understanding of the reasons for initial career choices, what prompted various job moves, what was learned from each, what was liked and so on. During this 'biographical review' a candidate will not only supply details of general work background but will also give hints about underlying attitudes, motivation and personality.

From this the interview should move to more direct concern with the vacant job. The intention is to get interviewees to talk about experiences that are directly relevant, rather than give theoretical answers to hypothetical questions, or prepared response to stock questions. Many interviews are spoilt by bombarding a candidate with direct and obvious questions in the early stages.

'Why do you want the job?' 'What skills have you that are relevant?' 'Why do you want to leave your present post?' Other common interviewing faults are the use of 'leading' questions, 'Obviously you enjoy that part of the work?' 'You are moving to gain wider experience?'; and an interviewer who talks, rather than asking simple questions and listening carefully to the response. This problem is probably caused by managers fearing an awkward silence in an interview. There are several ways of avoiding this. Preparation of a list of topics and a person specification checklist will provide prompts during the conversation. If this fails, an interviewer can summarise the last point made by a candidate to give time to think of the next question. Taking brief notes will give reminders of further information required. Note taking is also essential to assist recall after an interview. Clearly, this can distract the applicants, so a sensible balance is needed between making too few notes and spending too much time looking away from an interviewee whilst writing copious notes.

By relaxing but concentrating you will develop a free flowing interview. The aim should be for the candidate to talk for 80% of the time. If the structure of the interview is based on the outline we have suggested then the preliminary biographical review and specific questions about job experience and professional knowledge will take up three quarters of the time. At this point it is natural to provide more detailed information about the job, the unit, the hospital as well as the terms and conditions of employment. This leads to questions from the interviewee and then a conclusion in an encouraging and polite manner.

Immediately a candidate has left the room the interviewers should enlarge on their notes: to write up a more comprehensive interview report on the form prepared before the event. If this is left, it is likely that many facts and impressions will be forgotten after a series of interviews.

The final stage after all candidates have

been seen is to make a fair comparison between them and the main requirements of the job. Decisions not to appoint a shortlisted candidate should be based on a considered review of the value of her previous work experience, her standard of training, qualifications obtained, technical knowledge displayed, further study plans, attitudes towards the job, future career aspirations and practical circumstances. The quality of references should be taken into account as well as overall impressions of personal qualities. Care should be taken not to be too influenced by the actual interview performance or instinctive feelings of like and dislike towards the individual.

An interview should be a process of carefully building up information from a candidate that is relevant to the demands of the particular work situation, rather than an exercise in instant appraisal and personal bias.

PANEL INTERVIEWING

Potentially a panel of interviewers has several advantages over one-to-one interviewing. The individual bias and incompetence of individual panel members may be cancelled out. A well-balanced panel will be able to test more aspects of a candidate than a lone interviewer. All relevant technical and professional topics can be covered. It may be easier for individuals to listen and take notes whilst another asks questions. Applicants are more likely to get a comprehensive picture of a job and an organisation.

There are some drawbacks with this format. Most interviewees find the experience of facing four interviewers instead of one more intimidating. This increases the problem of self-confidence. Panel interviews are likely to be more formal in tone and favour the more extrovert applicant.

There are several fundamental considerations that can reduce the disadvantages and improve the value of the panel approach. Panel members should meet before the event to reach agreement on the key points of the person description for each vacancy. They should agree on how the interview will be conducted to obtain the relevant information and what information will be given to candidates. The members should act like a team as a result of this preparation. This will mean that they all show interest in questions being asked by other members and all listen to the replies from candidates. Within the panel structure it is usual to have a chairman to introduce and conclude the proceedings and to ensure that it goes according to plan. It is important that the direct supervisor of the vacant position is a member of the panel and plays a central part in the final decision. If interviews are to be used as the means of comparing different applicants for the same post it is important that each is given broadly similar interviews.

Given adequate preparation the actual approach is essentially the same for several people interviewing together as it is for an individual. They should go through the seven stages with the overall intention of engaging in free-flowing conversation about relevant topics. Greater effort will be needed to reduce the formality often associated with panel interviews. The main advantage of this format is in providing a more balanced and thorough assessment afterwards. Here again there must be effective teamwork and discipline. At the conclusion of each interview panel members should write up their notes in silence. The chairman should check whether all are satisfied with the amount of information obtained and the way that the *panel* conducted the interview. It is preferable not to exchange detailed opinions on candidate suitability until all interviews have been completed.

The NHS appointments procedures usually require references from previous employers or personal referees. There is debate about the value of such information and how it should be used. Some believe that a good reference indicates that an employer is pleased to lose the individual. This is much too cynical a view but it is likely that references will be too generalised to be really helpful and, whether good or bad, are only a reflection of one person's biased opinion of another. There is a dilemma in whether references should be read before an interview or left until assessments have been made by the selectors from their own opinions. It is probably better to leave them until the final stage of selection decision-making so that interviews are not influenced by preconceived views drawn from a possibly unfair reference.

Effectiveness as an interviewer in staff selection is not difficult to develop, provided adequate attention is given to preparation and that each interviewer has an awareness of the aims and skills involved in such conversations.

REFERENCES

Armstrong M 1985 Personnel practice, Kogan Page, London
Cumming M 1978 Personnel management in the National Health Service. Heinemann, London
Goodworth C 1983 Effective interviewing for employment selection. Business Books, London

19

Staff induction and training

Decisions on appointing or promoting staff are of great importance to the quality of health care. It is essential that even when care and appropriate techniques are employed managers should give proper attention to the introduction and training of a new member of staff so that she can soon become a fully integrated and effective employee.

It is useful to divide this into two tasks. The first is necessary for all staff from the most junior to the most highly skilled, or senior. This can be regarded as the initial induction and orientation to ensure that starters will apply their existing skills as soon as possible in the new environment. The second is further training and education to bring skills and knowledge to the level required to fill a role satisfactorily. Although some staff will be recruited who are adequately skilled, many actually take new jobs because they represent promotion or an opportunity to acquire wider experiences. Thus even qualified staff may benefit from some basic or refresher training.

INDUCTION

A considerable amount of information is needed before we can settle down in a new post. In simple jobs unfamiliarity with the new surroundings and ways of working can be rapidly overcome. In senior posts this induction period may last for several months.

163

A nurse manager should plan to meet the information needs of new staff quickly and in so doing help them overcome the anxiety which is often associated with joining a new unit. The planning process should start before new staff arrive. In this way a well-organised induction programme will result. Some senior nurses associate induction with a one or two-day course run by the school of nursing or other training staff. Although this can be incorporated into an induction programme, such courses are likely to be the least important aspect of acclimatisation.

New staff are most concerned about their immediate working colleagues and the details of their work tasks. First impressions of a unit are important therefore. It is encouraging to know that you are expected, that a plan has been formed of a systematic way to introduce you to the unit and that managers and staff are willing to give time and encouragement to someone new. Thus the most significant parts of induction are within the control of line managers and supervisors.

In carrying out this duty it is useful to consider three questions:

1. What information does a new entrant require to be able to settle down properly?
2. How can this information best be provided?
3. When can this information best be provided?

Precise information needs will vary according to the particular job, unit and the existing knowledge of the starter; but these items can all be identified under headings which are applicable anywhere. This induction checklist is often provided to section heads by personnel or training staff. If this is not the practice, line managers should devise their own. Some of the information on this list should be given during selection interviews and contained in a letter of appointment but it is wise to cover this again during the initial days in employment.

The methods available to provide induction information are:

— Staff handbook
— Appointment letter
— Personal talk with section head
— Tour of department
— Tour of unit
— Tour of hospital
— Procedure manuals — policy manuals
— Department records and files
— Talk with experienced senior staff
— Meeting with senior managers
— Introduction to other unit staff
— Maps
— Notices and memos
— Hospital induction/orientation course
— Video/film
— Self-teaching programme.

A comprehensive induction plan would use the appropriate resource to provide information in the order of most importance. It is usually a good policy to give a limited amount of information at a time, the exact opposite of some organisational practices of submitting starters to two or three days intensive orientation away from the job environment. Most new entrants are keen to meet work colleagues and get on with some practical work rather than sit through talks and films about safety procedures and District policies.

An example of an induction plan for night staff in a district general hospital combines a programme of familiarisation with a particular ward with attendance at the hospital's induction course. The complete process covers staff nurses, enrolled nurses, nursing auxiliaries and is the responsibility of the ward sister.

Sister greets newcomers, shows them round the ward and introduces them to other staff. Next she goes through an induction checklist indicating such key information as: contacting doctors, contacting sister, emergency procedures, fire drill, blood bank, theatre location, canteen location, working arrangements, rules, timesheets, off-duty book, request book. The policy and procedures book is shown which staff are asked to read at convenient moments; then they are attached to a senior member of staff to continue familiarisation more informally. Arrangements are made for staff to attend the two-day hospital induction course. Sisters have planned to extend this induction so that staff are also taken to other departments and understand procedures that have an impact on their own ward. This will be incorporated at convenient times in the first few weeks of employment.

As with all management activity it is necessary to monitor the progress of an induction programme. This can be accomplished by the use of a checklist, but more importantly by discussion with new employees. Line managers should carry out an informal induction interview at an appropriate time during the first few weeks to identify any problems affecting the new entrant and to evaluate the effectiveness of the induction programme.

An extension of this policy is that of carrying

Content	Responsible	Completed
1. Undertake a tour of the hospital		
2. Understand the internal telephone system and be able to utilise it		
3. Know how to bleep medical and nursing staff		
a. Know how to put out a crash call		
b. Know the location of the equipment		
c. Know the personnel involved and the routine		
4 Know the principles of the fire drill		
5. Subsequently attend a practice drill		
6. Know of the presence and location of policies and procedures. Ultimately have a working knowledge of them		
7. Have a broad outline of ward routine		
8. Have a working knowledge of the nursing observation charts		
9. Undertake a drug round with a senior member of nursing staff		
10. Possess a Control and Administration of Drugs Manual, initially with specific reference to:		
a. Controlled drug keys		
b. Medicine keys		
11. Be conversant with routine admissions		
12. Be conversant with emergency admissions		
13. Possess a major incident procedure book		
14. Attend a major incident seminar		
15. Attend an intravenous additives course		
16. Attain a proficiency certificate in intravenous additives		
17. Attend hospital induction programme		
18. Be conversant with procedure for booking annual leave		
19. Know where to find the list of off-duty staff		
20. Be conversant with procedure regarding accidents/incidents		
21. Be given knowledge or information sisters like to receive		
22. Know when to telephone a doctor		
23. Be conversant with hospital policy re sick leave and return to work		
24. Be conversant with meal break policy		
25. Have an understanding of students' expectations and concerns re night duty		
26. Have knowledge of hospital policy re uniforms		
27. Possess UKCC accountability leaflet and code of ethics.		

Fig. 19.1 Induction checklist.

out 'exit interviews' with staff who give notice to leave. The aim is to understand the reasons for leaving and to identify any aspects of employment experience that have been unsatisfactory. Where staff leave after a brief period of employment it is likely that a poor induction experience was a contributing factor. It can be useful also to ask existing staff for suggestions on improving the induction arrangements in a unit.

TRAINING

Training is the means by which staff acquire the level of knowledge and skills to perform their jobs satisfactorily. Therefore training is essential for all occupations. All managers should be interested in the quality of training offered to their staff. Within the NHS there is a great concern with preparing professional staff to meet the standards of education and training set by various professional bodies.

Passing professional examinations alone does not mean that individuals will be fully competent as practitioners. Further practical skills and knowledge are needed.

Nurse managers accept that they have an essential role in the professional training of student nurses and in assisting newly qualified staff to full professional competence. Yet problems of staff shortage in some wards and in the community services can force senior nurses to rely on students and inexperienced auxiliary staff to form an essential part of the nursing resource. This can mean a reduction in the quality of practical training provided. Despite the difficulties, it is important that senior nurses are able to make the most of the learning opportunities that are available for junior staff by an understanding of the procedures and skills employed in systematic training.

Systematic training

There are two ways for management to organise basic job training. One is to take on new staff, appoint them immediately to their post where the supervisor, or an experienced employee, will attempt to teach them how to tackle the job tasks. This is an 'informal' approach to training. Although it seems somewhat haphazard it is not necessarily inefficient, and in small organisations or with limited resources it may be the only practical system available. There are disadvantages in such a loosely structured approach however:

1. The training period is likely to be longer than necessary, as knowledge and skills are not learned systematically.
2. During the training period the performance of experienced staff and supervisors can be reduced as they provide guidance to trainees.
3. The knowledge and skills obtained in this informal way may not be the more desirable ones.
4. Trainees may become discouraged by the apparently random nature of their training.

The alternative way of training is based on a more considered and planned approach which could be regarded as 'systematic'.

In general the basic stages in this approach are:

1. Analyse the tasks to be learned. This requires a reliable job description indicating aims, duties and tasks. From this a 'skills analysis' can be produced listing the detailed knowledge and skills required to carry out these tasks and meet the aims.
2. Undertake a 'training needs analysis' of potential trainees. This involves assessing how much of the knowledge and skill indicated in the skills analysis is actually possessed by trainees. Tests and interviews can be used to make this judgement. If trainees' knowledge or skill is less than required a 'training need' will exist.
3. Prepare a 'training plan'. This is a systematic statement showing how the gaps in trainees' existing knowledge and skill can be met in the shortest time compatible with really learning the job and being cost effective.
4. Carry out the training, ensuring that those

required to provide instruction can do this adequately and that the training media is properly prepared and delivered.

5. Monitor the progress of the training programme to ensure it is carried out and to maintain the motivation of the trainee.
6. Evaluate the effectiveness of the training programme to check whether it did provide trainees with appropriate knowledge and skill, whether they are able to apply this in the work situation, whether they felt satisfied with the training, whether any aspects of the job are missed and how future training might be improved.

There are several applications of this planned approach to training for nurses. The overall scheme of professional nurse education aims to give new entrants a comprehensive and relevant grounding in general nursing theory and practice and then to provide additional specialist training. The structure of the scheme was reviewed in 1986, but proposed modifications will still retain the combination of 'off the job' education with 'on the job' practical training within the Health Service. The design of national professional qualification training will take account of the nature of knowledge and skills needed by practitioners, but will be more concerned with general grounding and considerations of developments in caring practices and medical technology, than locally based training aimed at practical skills development for learners or at upgrading skills of newly recruited staff in current procedures.

It is important to evaluate all forms of training to ensure that they are an integral part of an overall 'manpower plan'. This requires corporate level management to identify the future shape of the service and the nature of staff needed to provide it.

Health authority planning at national and then regional level is a complex task, but expressed simply it depends on having information to make predictions on future demand for health care (size of population, age profiles, expectations, disease trends, birth rates etc.), information to assess the required manpower resources to provide service at various levels of demand and expectation (size of workforce now, distribution amongst occupational groups, age profile, wastage rates, recruitment patterns etc.), added to possible advances in technology and medicine which affect layout and skill requirements.

At district level the same analysis will be required but on a smaller scale, whilst taking account of national policies. As a result of redistribution of resources from central London health authorities during the 1980s to more outlying districts, some authorities have started building programmes to extend health care provision. This will require management to consider whether additional staff will be required, whether these could be recruited locally, what training will be needed, whether existing staff will need additional training to cope with different specialities or to fill senior posts. A budget will be needed to ensure that training is carried out so that the additional services are properly manned.

Thus training at ward level can be short term to bring the members of the ward team up to basic standards and part of a long-term plan to ensure that staff are available to replace leavers, staff new services and cope with changes in patient care.

We have outlined six basic stages in a systematic approach to training.

We shall now examine three aspects in greater detail — making training plans, delivering training and training evaluation.

Training plans

All successful training requires motivated trainees and a completely organised training programme. A student should know what she can expect to learn in a particular ward and the ward sister should be aware of what the student needs to learn. If these two perceptions coincide after discussion, then when a student arrives on a ward it is likely that enthusiasm will be engendered. This will be maintained if subsequent learning experiences meet expectations.

Planning by sisters can start with a list of

learning opportunities — patients nursed, medicine and drugs used in treatment, nursing procedures performed. The list can be incorporated into a bar chart plan (see Ch. 5) with the students and the main learning experiences displayed. This gives students confidence that they will benefit from training, and enables the sister to control training in an efficient manner.

This indicates 'what' will be learned. The second step should clarify 'how' this will be learned. It is unfortunate that 'learning' for many people still implies having a teacher and lessons. Yet there is a great variety of learning methods which can be used, especially in the practical situations of 'on the job' training in health care.

Learning can be generally defined as meaning any experience which results in a more or less permanent change in individual behaviour.

In this context 'behaviour' means any difference in a person which may include the ability to talk or write about facts, use manual skills, operate new equipment, follow procedures etc., but it is not possible to know whether learning has taken place unless tangible change in behaviour can be identified.

Unfortunately there is no universally accepted 'learning theory', although some authorities have put forward general, common sense principles of learning. The theoretical background to the acquisition of skill has been concerned with a study of the process by which we learn new behaviour in response to specific inputs of information. The pattern of response (R) to a specific stimulus (S) has evolved in the S–R theory of learning. Thus, in learning to drive a car we learn a chain of stimuli and responses, such as changing speed of the engine (stimulus) and the need to change gear (response).

It is too simple to consider all learning as a chain of stimulus and response as there are other factors involved. One of these is the spontaneous acquisition of certain skills due to processes within the individual not directly related to a gradual build-up of correct responses to specific stimuli. In training of more complex perceptual skill, as opposed to motor skills, the S–R theory again is not fully applicable. Despite the theoretical problems, it is possible to put forward guidelines that could be used to make learning more effective for adults in work.

Learning is likely to occur most readily where the following conditions are fulfilled:

1. The skills and knowledge to be taught are understood by the trainer before training begins.
2. The present skills and knowledge of trainees are known by the trainer before training begins.
3. The learning moves from the limit of existing skill and knowledge into new areas.
4. The existing attitudes of trainees to training, the job and the organisation are known by the trainer before training begins.
5. The abilities of trainees are known by the trainer.
6. The trainees are reasonably motivated in general towards training ('over-motivation' may create learning problems, especially when difficulties are experienced by the trainee as anxiety may result).
7. The trainees are reasonably motivated towards the specific skills they are to learn. This will be better where the motivation is intrinsic (because of extra pay etc.).
8. Reasonable and realistic targets are set which are meaningful to the trainee.
9. Knowledge of results is given frequently to individual trainees.
10. Desirable responses to training are reinforced and key factors are emphasised with backing up and reinforcement.
11. Good performances by trainees are positively rewarded rather than mistakes being punished, as a means of giving knowledge of results.
12. Appropriate prompting and correction are given so that trainees are able to perform new skills with success.
13. Failures and mistakes by trainees are

compensated by successful experience in training.

14. Trainees take an active part in the training rather than passively receive instructions.
15. Meaningful practice is set, and the spacing of practice periods is effective for the skills being learned.
16. Length of instruction and practice periods are not too great.
17. Instructions and lectures are given in clear positive language.
18. The transfer of learning in the training situation to the requirements of the real job is made easier by training exercises using the same or similar materials etc.
19. The training environment is reasonably good.
20. There are good, friendly relationships between trainees.
21. There is a good relationship between the instructors and the trainees.
22. The expectations of trainees about training are broadly in line with the realities of training.
23. The expectations of trainees about the real work situation are in line with the realities of the situation.
24. The results of previous training are evaluated and methods are modified in the light of properly acquired judgements of past results.

As skill in work, whether as a manager, a nurse, a porter or an administrator, depends on an individual recognising and understanding information that is presented by his environment and acting in an appropriate manner in response to this, training is concerned with enabling individuals to recognise and interpret information and to make specific responses.

Training methods

Traditional methods of teaching have concentrated largely on the spoken word supported by additional visual material. In broad terms, people find it easier to assimilate new information and to understand new situations the

more senses that come into play during the learning and the more they are able to take an active rather than a passive part.

The range of training methods that can be used by nurse managers, either in the role of full-time tutor or for on-the-job instruction for junior staff, is quite wide.

Lectures and talks

This method has considerable advantages, as well as significant drawbacks. Where a group of people need specific information which is capable of simple logical presentation, then the lecture is an excellent means of giving them this information.

A lecture, even on suitable subjects, will vary in effectiveness according to the skill of the lecturer. There are a number of simple points which can improve the quality of a verbal presentation, but giving all but short talks is a skilled occupation requiring considerable practice. The points which can help a talk are:

1. The content should be carefully planned.
2. The language used should be appropriate to the audience's existing knowledge and attitudes.
3. The lecture should follow a clear, logical sequence.
4. The audience should be made aware of the overall structure of the lecture.
5. The main points should be reinforced.
6. Visual aids, such as blackboards, posters, slides etc., should be used but not overdone.
7. The voice should be used so that everyone can hear easily, and concentration is made easy by varying the material, pace and manner of delivery. Humour can help in this respect.
8. The lecture should run to a time scheme based on the principle that talking for twenty minutes without a break is the maximum that even keen and able listeners should be expected to sustain. The maximum is reduced for a less interested or able audience.

9. Questions and participation should be encouraged within the framework of the lecture.
10. Notes, references and reading material should be provided.

The same principles and problems emerge when verbal instruction is used as part of a practical demonstration.

Obviously, demonstrations should quickly lead to practice on the part of the trainee, supported by constructive help and criticism by the instructor.

Discussions

Many formal lectures end in general discussion and obviously there are many advantages in getting a group to ask questions of the lecturer and other people in the group. This is especially useful where subjects are of a controversial nature, and where individuals in the group find their existing ideas have been challenged. It is extremely difficult to change individual attitudes and a formal talk is unlikely to achieve change. Reaction from a group of peers may be more influential in altering a person's view of a subject.

Discussion groups can be used as a means of learning without a formal lecture at all. To be effective the leader needs as much skill as that required to present an effective lecture. The leader needs to ensure that:

1. There is enough material to arouse discussion.
2. The group provides as many answers as possible.
3. The discussion is gently guided along desired lines.
4. All members participate.
5. Conclusions and summary of main points are made.

Simulation exercises

The disadvantages of lectures and discussions are that the ideas and information presented may not be transferred to the real job situation. To assist transfer a variety of simulation exercises are used in skills training, such as practice with a dummy during first aid instruction.

It is important that the skills learned under simulated conditions are the same as the skills needed on the job, otherwise transference of learning may be hindered.

There are obviously greater problems involved in simulating social administration and management situations in the training environment. There are available means of doing this to a limited extent through case studies, case histories, in-tray exercises, role playing, incident examination and games.

The objective in this method is to provide trainees with background facts of a situation (problem of staff discipline, patient complaints about treatment etc.), then either ask trainees to decide on the action they would take in the circumstances, or to comment on the actions.

The presentation of the case can be verbal, in writing, by film or video recordings. Case studies can be used by individual trainees, or by groups.

Case studies have the advantages of getting participation of trainees and of getting them to consider 'real' problems.

In this respect trainees' own experiences can be used as the basis for 'live' case studies.

The aim of using 'in tray' exercises is to place trainees in pressurised situations in which they have to read a number of items, make decisions on the items and write notes, reports, memoranda or letters containing these decisions. Obviously a great deal of background information is given as well, so that the trainee will be familiar with the organisation in which the exercise is set. She will be expected to use previously learned information and techniques as well.

Role playing requires trainees to improvise parts in a scene which require the use of skills and knowledge that are relevant to the job being learned (encounters between nurses and a patient's relatives, handling complaints from a shop steward etc.). A scenario can be prepared by a trainer. Alternatively, actual problems that trainees have encountered in work can be built up in to a role playing exercise during a training session.

Learning in all such activities will be facilitated by detailed briefing after the event. This is best approached by encouraging participants to discuss what happened in the exercise and to identify significant learning points. The trainer can identify additional points missed. The use of questionnaires or video recording can aid this learning analysis.

The most ambitious simulation exercises are games. In these full business, professional or administrative activities may be simulated so that participants have enough information on processes, finance, supplies, staffing and resources to be able to make decisions.

The main advantage of games is that the outcome of the decisions can be fed back to the participants quickly so the experience of making decisions on a long-term scale can be condensed into a few hours. Another characteristic of games can be their interactive nature. That is, where a decision is made by one group it will influence the total situation (share of budget etc.) and thus a further dimension in the decision-making process is learned.

Discovery learning

Active participation of trainees can be encouraged by exercises requiring them to find out things for themselves. Observing a nursing procedure and writing a report on what happened, researching a topic for presentation to other trainees, or visiting another unit with the task of obtaining specific information are examples of 'discovery learning'.

Film and video

There is an extensive range of filmed material available for all types of training. Films are popular for the entertainment elements, but are often too general and are essentially a passive form of learning. They are useful to introduce, or reinforce, learning points.

The development of cheap video recorders and cameras means that organisations can make their own training programmes. These can be more specific than professionally produced films. Recording can also be made of training activities or of real working activities. These can be played back and used for coaching. This is a very powerful training method but it must be used with care as there is a danger of undermining the confidence of trainees by emphasising their faults.

Audio tapes

There is greater demand on a listener listening to a tape than on a viewer watching a film, but this can make it an effective learning method. A substantial library of audio material is available for training and educational purposes.

Programmed learning

These learning methods are basically 'self-learning'. By use of a text, a teaching machine or interactive video a student is presented with small items of information and then given multiple choice questions. The intention is that the learner should make the right choice most of the time, and thus reinforce the item before moving to the next.

This technique requires a very careful preparation of the material but has the advantage of removing the need for an instructor and ensuring that individuals go through each item, at their own pace.

Another means of getting trainees to take an active part in the learning process is to set specific items to read and questions about the items.

Distance learning

For many years people have studied for professional qualification by correspondence courses involving reading prepared material and submitting written work for assessment. The Open University extended this concept to include teaching by use of self-study booklets, guided reading, TV, video, and audio tapes. During the 1980s there have been considerable extensions of this technique into many other aspects of professional training,including nursing and other health care occupations. The advantages of distance learning are that trainees can work at their own pace, at times convenient to them and with less time away from their work. The disadvantages are that a learner may become demotivated from the isolation and problems of keeping up with a study schedule, or because materials are not directly relevant. It is likely, however, that more professional training will be available in distance learning formats as it is convenient and generally more economic for employers.

Evaluating training

All training programmes should be reviewed and evaluated to assess: (a) the skill level reached by trainees, (b) the time taken to achieve this, (c) the cost involved, (d) possible improvements in future training, and (e) relevance or transference to the real job situation.

There are a number of ways of attempting these evaluations. The simplest is an objective test at the end of a training programme or after each section, to find the extent to which the new knowledge and skills have been learned by the trainee. These tests could be practical (operating a machine, filling in a form, emergency procedures etc.) or in the form of a written test. Assuming that the trainee did not have any knowledge of the subject before the course, this is an evaluation of the learning.

In addition to seeking to determine what has been learned, the trainer can find out how much trainees feel they have learned, how valuable they found this and how useful they feel it will be to them. This enquiry can be made at the end of training or sometimes later or at both times.

Testing how much of the information that has been presented in training has been learned by the trainee does not necessarily mean that this learning will be applied in the job, or that this has been relevant to the job.

In practical jobs, quantified information on job performance can usually be obtained. In the case of administrative and supervisory jobs this is much more difficult. Here the trainer can ask the individuals who have been through the training programme the extent to which they feel training has improved their performance. The trainer can ask the immediate superior to assess work standards. Obviously all these enquiries should be conducted in as objective a manner as possible.

Thus there are five areas in which assessment can be made of the value of a training programme.

1. How much more knowledge and skill trainees have at the end of the programme than before they started.
2. How much extra knowledge and skill trainees feel that they have obtained.
3. How relevant they feel this is to their job.
4. How relevant the knowledge and skill really is to the job.
5. How relevant the line management feel the training programme has been to job performance.

Management training

Although some improvements could be made in the training of nursing staff, generally the NHS has an excellent record of concern and investment in professional education for nurses, both at basic and updating levels. Such a judgement does not extend to the record on management training.

In the 1970s an effort was made to overcome this problem by a framework of 'off the job' foundation and specialist management courses. It is not possible to learn to be a good manager simply by attending a short course and often too much is expected from such training. There should be a planned programme of basic management training for all staff immediately preceding or shortly after promotion to a post of supervisory responsibility.

The responsibilty for ensuring that all managers and supervisors in a hospital or health care service are properly trained rests with senior line management. General managers of units and services should regard this of prime importance. Within the nursing service, again the responsibility should be accepted by the most senior nurse manager. Too often management training is left to training staff who may lack seniority and credibility. Line managers should take advice on the best means of providing effective training but should not delegate the overall responsibility.

In trying to ensure that newly promoted or appointed managers are given appropriate training, it is possible to apply a similar systematic approach that can be used in operative and basic professional training. The starting point should be an assessment of the skill and knowledge content of a nurse management post and then an appraisal of the post-holder to identify knowledge and skill needs. A training plan can then be devised using the range of training media and on-the-job coaching (see the next chapter) appropriate to the training needs. This scheme should be supplemented by attendance at appropriate courses available within an authority, provided by local colleges and by independent management training organisations.

The progress of individuals through this scheme should be monitored by periodic discussion and assessment of job performance. In this way the training is evaluated and can be continually improved.

Managing, like nursing and medicine, is not an art which you can simply learn and then become a fully competent practitioner. All managers need to consider how to advance beyond a basic level of expertise, and how to keep abreast of the many changes that affect their role.

An effective manager is one who is engaged in continuous learning for continuing self-development, and is encouraging towards more junior staff so that they have learning opportunities to aid their professional and personal development. We consider the techniques and problems of staff and management development in the next chapter.

REFERENCES

Coutts L, Hardy L 1985 Teaching for health. Churchill Livingstone, Edinburgh
Ewan C, White R 1984 Teaching nursing. Croom Helm, London
Fretwell J 1982 Ward teaching and learning, RCN, London
Gott M 1984 Learning nursing, RCN, London
Orton H 1981 Ward learning climate, RCN, London

20
Staff development

It is difficult to make a precise distinction between the concepts involved in staff training and those of staff development — there is only a different emphasis. Training is an activity which provides learning relevant to basic competence in a role, while development is concerned with learning beyond the basics. Staff with aspirations towards professionalism need to improve upon their present performance and keep pace with the advances in their profession. This implies that all senior staff in health care should subscribe to the idea of being 'self-developing'.

Health care organisations cannot rely on the development efforts of individual staff, however; there must be an overall policy to meet three main purposes: one is to ensure that the services provided do keep abreast of advanced concepts and techniques of medicine; the second is to encourage staff to seek improvements to their job performance, even if it is already at an acceptable level; the third is to ensure that staff with most potential are prepared for greater responsibility, thus ensuring a smooth succession as senior staff retire or move on.

Many organisations in this country, both public service and profit making, have failed to provide sufficient resources for staff and career development. Often senior managers feel that they have made it to the top largely by their own efforts, therefore the next generation should follow the same process. When senior posts become vacant there is often a preference to fill them from outside.

The NHS has certainly lacked a coherent programme of career development for nurses so that the majority of general manager appointments during 1985/6 were filled by managers from a non-nursing background. Since then the NHS training authority has advocated a more systematic system of development of potential senior managers.

It is unfortunate, however, if development is considered only in association with promotion. Many organisations have been forced to reduce the numbers employed in managerial and senior specialist positions, thus reducing promotion opportunities. At the same time, organisations need to generate a desire for excellence and innovation amongst staff. Thus there is a need for 'continuous learning' as a means of organisational development and survival. For individuals, development should be an end in itself. Learning more, using greater skill and helping others to improve, will increase your satisfaction with work —

meeting some of your self-actualisation needs.

Who should be responsible for staff development? If development is a necessary part of the continued improvement or survival of an organisation, then all managers should be responsible for initiating their own development and devising development plans for their staff. In practice, such a developmental culture needs encouragement and resourcing by the most senior levels of management.

Equally, if development is associated with career and succession planning then, although the detailed application of a scheme can be carried out by personnel or training staff, endorsement must come from senior line management. Meeting the organisational and personal aims of development requires a variety of activities. These can be summarised in Figure 20.1.

The review stage involves some form of staff appraisal/self-appraisal/peer assessment/team review which should lead to identifying aspects of present performance to improve

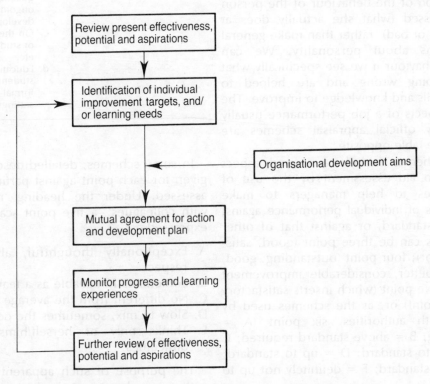

Fig. 20.1 The staff development process.

and actions which could assist promotion prospects.

APPRAISAL SCHEMES

All managers make assessments of the quality of their subordinates (as well as colleagues and senior staff), but these judgements can be unfair and of limited practical use. Senior nurses may consider various nurses as 'doing really well', 'needs to improve her attitude' or 'will be lucky to ever get promotion'. These are personal opinions that give no tangible evidence of the specific strengths and weaknesses, or indications of how improvements could be made.

Many organisations including health authorities have introduced systems to help managers make fairer and more detailed assessments of subordinates. A few also encourage peer assessment, team appraisals and self-assessment. The conventional schemes require a line manager, as appraiser, to give detailed consideration of the behaviour of the person to be assessed (what she actually does at work, good or bad), rather than make general observations about personality. We can improve behaviour if we see specifically what we are doing wrong and are helped to develop skills and knowledge to improve. The specific aspects of a job performance usually covered by official appraisal schemes are listed in the table opposite.

Many schemes include a second aspect intended to aid assessment by the use of rating scales to help managers to make comparisons of individual performance against a defined standard, or against that of other staff. Scales can be three point (good, satisfactory, poor); four point (outstanding, good, could be better, considerable improvement needed); five point (which inserts satisfactory as a mid-point) or, as the schemes used by some health authorities, six point (A = outstanding; B = above standard required; C = well up to standard; D = up to standard; E = below standard; F = definitely not up to standard)

General factors found in appraisal schemes	Factors found in appraisal schemes for nursing staff

1. Quality of work produced
2. Quantity of work produced
3. Job and task knowledge
4. Time keeping
5. Attendance
6. Initiatives
7. Decision-making
8. Delegation
9. Organisational ability
10. Leadership of section
11. Co-operation with others
12. Administration skills
13. Written and verbal skills
	1. Organisation and management of work.
	2. Supervision of staff and leadership
	3. Relationships
	  a. with patients
	  b. with immediate colleagues: medical; administrative; ancillary and other groups of staff
	  c. with social services departments, schools and supportive agencies
	  d. with nursing management
	  e. with learners, visiting lecturers and other visitors
	4. Ability to communicate;
	  a. in writing
	  b. orally
	5. Teaching and training:
	  a. patients and their relatives etc. (e.g. health education)
	  b. qualified staff (e.g. in ongoing on-the-job development)
	  c. On the job training of students/pupils etc.
	  d. Education of students/pupils in formal and informal settings

In some schemes, detailed descriptions are given for each point against particular factors assessed. Under the heading 'relationships with colleagues', a five point scale could be expressed as:

A. Exceptionally thoughtful, always gains respect
B. Sometimes noticeable as a team member
C. No different from the average
D. Slow to mix, sometimes the odd one out
E. Thinks only of herself/himself, causes difficulties.

The purpose of such apparently elaborate systems can be summarised as:

1. Encourages appraiser to be fair and specific in reviewing subordinates
2. Gives comparative assessments year by year and a record of improvement
3. Forms the basis of a constructive discussion between appraiser and appraisee
4. Assists with the planning of training and other development events.

The theory underlying appraisal seems constructive and essential to any progressive organisation. There are practical problems, however, which have led some formal appraisal schemes to be abandoned or discredited. Some of these difficulties are:

1. Lack of direct knowledge by appraiser of the appraisee's real job performance and potential, either because they do not share the same professional background or because there is too little contact between them.
2. Poor relationships between appraiser and appraisee making constructive discussion difficult.
3. Lack of commitment by appraiser to the concept of staff development.
4. Lack of commitment by appraisee to concept of staff development.
5. Lack of organisational resources to provide agreed action plans.
6. Poor interviewing skill by appraiser
7. Scheme may be linked to awarding pay increases, thus inhibiting appraisee from accepting weaknesses in performance.
8. Scheme may be seen as linked with promotion which again can inhibit frank discussions.

The most serious obstacle to useful appraisal is the lack of commitment by a senior nurse who does not believe in the value of open review and positive development.

APPRAISAL INTERVIEWING

A properly conducted official appraisal meeting should in itself be a valuable learning experience, both for the senior nurse and the member of staff.

Unfortunately, the model used by many managers is basically authoritarian. The manager is a judge, the subordinate is the judged, so that criticism or praise which has been written onto an appraisal form is simply read aloud. The subordinate either accepts the judgement, signs the appraisal form and ends the encounter, or seeks to defend himself against unfair criticism. In either event little learning will take place, and little of practical consequence follows.

Appraisal interviews should be based on a more participative model. The manager needs to accept the value of a two-way discussion where a sister can get some feedback from a staff nurse and an assessment of her own performance and where she might reconsider her own opinions of the staff nurse's work and so end with mutual commitment to improve.

If a manager accepts this concept, the actual planning and conduct of the interview will be easy. If the basic attitude is unsympathetic, the interview will either be superficial or a defensive conversation.

Formal appraisal should be a supplement to regular informal individual coaching and assessment and self-appraisal. Real development will not flourish from an annual appraisal alone. Thus in discussing the conduct of appraisal interviews we shall also consider the wider question of coaching and counselling.

Preparation

It is certainly necessary to give thought to an appraisal/coaching interview before the event, but there is a danger that excessive preparation will make the meeting too one-sided. Thus a disadvantage of the appraisal form, especially in giving such apparently precise grades as C, D etc., is that the decisions made by the appraiser/coach will leave little scope for open discussion at the interview.

Ideally, as interviewer you should identify particular points for praise and, if applicable, points of concern, with specific examples to support criticism of your subordinate.

The appraisee should be given notice of the proposed meeting, which should be held at a convenient time in a suitably private location, free from interruptions. In formal schemes a blank appraisal form is usually issued so that the subordinate can attempt some self-appraisal by way of preparation. For more informal coaching, little if any preparation by staff is needed, or desirable.

Interviewing skills

In the sections concerning communication (Ch. 10) and counselling (Ch. 16) we have given detailed guidance on interviewing techniques which will be equally relevant to coaching/appraisal. In many respects, however, the term 'interview' is inappropriate; frank and constructive discussion is the ideal to be achieved. Thus there is a need to use open questions, to probe for deeper understanding of the subordinates' views, and to listen carefully whilst trying to keep a relaxed atmosphere. If, as 'coach', you simply tell others your views of their shortcomings, even expressed in friendly and helpful terms, it is likely that they will experience this as criticism and will become defensive, or will listen politely but will not change their behaviour in practice.

A specific formula which seeks to avoid these problems and has been well tested in practice is given below:

1. Introduction

Try to outline the purpose of the 'interview' in a positive way, avoiding the impression that it is criticism or discipline but more to do with training and development. Try to get the respondent to express reactions to this so that misunderstandings and fears can be removed at the beginning.

2. Check job objectives, priorities and job description

If this is the first coaching/appraisal session, try to get the respondent to explain how she sees the job — what it involves and what are the main priorities — and compare this with the official job description and your views.

If previous discussions about the job have been undertaken it is still appropriate to check the validity of the job description.

3. Seek 'subordinate's' view of performance and career aspirations

If this is the first session, try to get the respondent to explain what she sees as good aspects of her current achievements and approaches. It would be helpful to confirm her views if you agree. Then seek a similar discussion about aspects for improvements, areas of lower achievements and difficulties encountered in trying to do a good job. If there have been previous interviews you should seek the respondent's views about progress achieved on improvement targets and any training received, before looking for further development needs.

4. Discuss 'superior's' view of subordinate's performance

From an understanding of how the respondent feels about the job, her achievements and problems, it should be possible to offer confirmation if you agree with this analysis. If there are points of disagreement or aspects missing these can be introduced in a constructive way for examination. It is usually advisable to start with points of praise rather than the less satisfactory aspects. Remember to have facts available to support your judgements.

5. Seek an 'action plan' from subordinate to improve performance

If some agreement has been reached on the points for improvement in present job performance then you should ask the subordinate for suggestions on how to improve her behaviour or achievements. If this is forthcoming you can reinforce the ideas that are appropriate and add further suggestions. It may be necessary to offer advice or to conduct a brief training session on how improvement might be achieved. (Alternatively this session could be arranged for a later date.)

6. Agree on specific objectives

Try to avoid having a list of generalised 'new year resolutions', but have new specific, attainable targets which the subordinate can commit herself to achieve within a set time-scale. In subsequent coaching sessions the 'interview' can follow the same pattern but will concentrate on a review of achievements in these particular targets. The structure is not intended as a rigid agenda to be followed in

---

Coaching — Specific periods set aside for 'coach' (who may be the immediate superior or someone with higher professional status) and staff or 'tutorials' to discuss matters which could improve the individuals skill's and knowledge.

Team meeting — Specific sessions for teams of staff to discuss matters which could improve their collective approach and competence.

Job enlargement — Delegating tasks, giving some job rotation, extending a role, standing in and acting up are all means to give an individual further opportunities for practical learning.

Projects — Giving individuals practical research either on managerial, administrative, technical or professional topics.

Action groups — Setting up small project groups, either departmental or interdepartmental, to conduct similar research and to experience further team working skills.

Secondments — Temporary move to another job inside an organisation, or with another employer. This can involve job swops.

Visits — Spending limited time in other departments or other organisations to obtain additional information and appreciation.

Courses — Attending 'in house' or external training courses relevant to specific learning needs.

Distance learning — Following a specific course through a distance learning method, or undertaking a programme of guided reading.

(There should be proper briefing and debriefing of staff experiences in any development activity.)

Fig. 20.2 Components of a development action plan.

all coaching sessions but as a suggested framework for those with limited experience.

7. Promotion aims

The discussion can then move to considerations of aspirations about the future. Again seek to understand the subordinates' thoughts; encourage these if appropriate or test the realism of their aims. Ideally there should be mutual agreement on actions that would enhance prospects for promotion.

It is important to take notes and make a record of points agreed. The final assessment on the official appraisal form can then be completed and agreed in the case of an appraisal interview.

Development action plan

The outcome of this review phase of a development activity could be improved motivation, closer relationships, clearer understanding of some problems and some additional factual information. There should also be a plan of action which will promote further learning. As adults in work we learn skills and acquire knowledge from a variety of experiences and information sources. These can be used in a deliberate way instead of relying on random opportunities or regarding formal training courses as the only means of development (see Fig. 20.2)

PROBLEMS WITH STAFF DEVELOPMENT

It is difficult to object to the theory of staff development in a service that depends on committed and competent staff who are ever willing to apply the outcome of research for the benefit of patients. In practice there are many factors which can inhibit staff development.

To have many staff following ambitious action plans implies that an organisation has spare capacity. This will be necessary if staff are to be absent on study days, working in project teams, attending meetings etc., whilst someone else covers the normal work load. Even if such cover is organised on the basis of development for those standing in, it will not work with staffing at minimum levels. Within the NHS of the 1980s there have been ward closures and service reductions from lack of funds. In these circumstances it can be difficult to devise staff development activities on the necessary scale.

Development does require effort on the part of the person going through the learning experience. This implies willingness and enthusiasm. Unfortunately, there is an alternative interpretation of a management which asks staff to take on extended duties, to stand in for absent colleagues and to undertake extra study without extra pay — it can be seen as exploitation. In parts of the NHS experienced staff will have reached the limit of their career ambitions, and whilst being prepared to be responsible in a role, will not be prepared to take on anything else.

Another attitude which is in conflict with the development idea is that which equates the need to learn with weakness, instead of being a positive act. Thus managers will be reluctant to accept criticism from their seniors, let alone openly admit to weakness or ignorance, or be prepared to seek critical feedback from junior staff, or managers in other departments.

This outlook will also present barriers to other managers or junior staff who wish to widen their knowledge through visits, coaching and open discussion.

MANAGEMENT DEVELOPMENT

In Chapter 19 we considered that basic training for management could be planned and executed using similar methodology to that applied to basic professional and technical training. Similarly, the concept of development beyond the basics and of continuous learning and a continuous search for excellence applies as much to managers as to professional staff.

It is useful to identify three aspects of planned management development. Each manager should be following a programme of personal development, based on the model of appraisal to diagnose development needs and to agree a multifarious development action plan; similarly separate management teams should be engaged in programmes of team improvement, whilst all management and senior staff development should be co-ordinated towards the goal of overall organisational development.

The choice of development methods employed for management development are of considerable importance. The traditional modes of instruction may be suitable for presenting fresh information on the technical aspects of management (appreciation of budgeting control, employment legislation, computer applications etc.), but are ineffective in improving interpersonal skills, decision-making, communication or coping with team work problems. Methods here should focus on the actual managers/supervisors and their existing behaviours and attitudes (being 'student centred' rather than 'trainer centred'). There should be examination of actual problems they encounter, or are expected to encounter ('problem centred') and engagement in activities where they can learn from experience.

This learning should be translated into effective management action thereafter ('action centred' and 'experiential learning').

CONCLUSIONS

If staff development, management development and organisational development are to flourish, the full support of review managers and the services of professional training facilitators are essential. The short-term appointments of general managers in the NHS, the emphasis on cost reduction and the generally low status of the personnel function suggest this idea will be difficult to achieve.

Despite these difficulties it is essential that a senior nurse who wishes to become fully competent in the management skills of her role, should adopt a developmental outlook, adapting the process for her own self-development whilst doing what she can to encourage subordinate staff, colleagues and more senior managers to display a similar outlook.

REFERENCES

Boyell T, Pedler M 1981 Management self development. Gower, Aldershot
Randell G, Packard P 1984 Staff appraisal. Institute of Personnel Management, Oxford
Singer E 1974 Effective management coaching, Institute of Personnel Management, Oxford

FOUR

Management techniques and health care

21
Managing industrial relations

There are several features of an organisation which have a significant influence on the role and effectiveness of line managers but over which they have little control. Within the NHS the terms and conditions of employment for staff and the definition of what constitutes satisfactory standards of staff conduct are matters for negotiation between representatives of several trade unions or professional associations, and the representatives of the service. As the outcome of these negotiations and the general quality of relationships with trade unions have a bearing on hours staff work, tasks they will undertake, and the disciplinary procedures available, nurse managers at ward level should have an informed interest in 'industrial relations' (IR).

What is industrial relations?

Many people associate the term with strikes and similar disruptive actions, but these situations are really a breakdown of industrial relations. In a practical sense industrial relations is part of organisational management that is concerned with creating the right circumstances that will ensure work is carried out in a productive manner. The achievement of this aim requires five essential conditions to be met in an organisation:

1. A framework of agreed terms and conditions of employment that are fair both to employees and to the employer

2. A framework of procedures to deal with disputes and problems concerning conditions of employment or working practices so that these are resolved without disruption
3. A system of effective communication and consultation between management and the work force
4. Managers who are competent in developing and maintaining co-operative working relations with their immediate work group, with trade union representatives and with other managers
5. Managers who are able to resolve IR problems effectively, using appropriate procedures.

Managing industrial relations is a broad task which is concerned with all matters that influence whether people will work in a productive manner. Thus the terms 'employee relations' or 'labour relations' can also be used.

Judging the quality of an organisation's labour relations will depend on where you are sitting. A regional personnel manager may consider the absence of strikes or other disruptive actions together with a reasonable level of co-operation from trade union officials as good features. The maintenance officer in a hospital might be more concerned about the backing he gets from his more senior managers when faced with shop floor problems. The shop steward would take account of the level of trade union membership, the level of consultation with local managers as well as the terms and conditions of employment whilst the average employee, whether in a hospital or a more commercial organisation, is likely to be interested in the level of take home pay compared to the amount of effort put in and compared with the earnings of other employees. Thus individuals drawn from different parts of the same district health authority will have different views about industrial relations, as they use different criteria to make their assessments, as well as having different experiences at work.

Despite these different perceptions it is possible to make some general observations about the quality of employee relations. From the management view as a whole, the factors of concern should be the level of work efficiency achieved by all sections of the work force (costs, outputs, quantity, quality, overheads etc.) and the amount of co-operation displayed by the work force and any of their representatives. It could be possible for general management to be satisfied with the level of efficiency, but feel that the amount of argument and dispute involved in achieving it is unacceptable and self-defeating in the long term. Alternatively, it could be considered that an organisation had generally pleasant relationships between staff and management but there was an urgent need to raise the level of efficiency. Clearly, it is not sensible to describe any organisation as having 'good' or 'bad' industrial relations. It is more appropriate for top management to consider whether the current balance between efficiency and co-operation could be improved, or has been deteriorating compared with other times or other organisations. In this case the state of IR health may be diagnosed as 'could be better' or alternatively 'satisfactory for the moment'.

Who is responsible for developing satisfactory employee relations? All health care managers have some responsibility reflecting their seniority and the amount of direct influence they have on sections of the work force. As most nurse managers work close to the point of health care delivery they have a particularly important role. The main aims of senior nurses in this task should be:

1. To provide appropriate leadership to all members of an immediate work group so that these staff feel motivated to work productively and behave in a co-operative manner
2. To resolve any problems that do arise within the group in a constructive manner using appropriate procedures and conforming to the authority rules and policies
3. To make appropriate representations to higher management and personnel staff to

obtain improvements in facilities, work arrangements and communication for section staff
4. To develop constructive relationships with shop stewards and to encourage them to act constructively within procedures
5. To seek advice and guidance from personnel and industrial relations staff when appropriate.

These aims are simple and would probably be acceptable by most senior nurses. Achieving them in practice can be a different matter. Many line managers in middle or junior posts find a number of difficulties that prevent them filling a really positive role in industrial relations matters. These problems, which are as likely to affect ward sisters as factory supervisors, can be summarised as:

— Junior managers lack information about changes in organisational policies and conditions.
— Junior managers have little influence or credibility with their more senior managers.
— Junior managers are not consulted about IR matters by higher managers, or personnel specialists.
— Junior managers receive little backing in dealing with IR problems and will have their authority undermined by higher managers.
— Higher managers consult directly with Shop Stewards.
— Shop stewards have special relationships with personnel/industrial relations managers.
— Employees take their problems to shop stewards rather than their own supervisors.
— Shop stewards have more information about conditions, procedures, policies and changes than junior managers.
— Shop stewards are seen by staff as having more influence to get things done than junior managers.
— Some shop stewards do not follow procedures and encourage staff to be uncooperative with junior managers.
— Junior managers have poor facilities and limited opportunities to communicate with their staff.
— There is a considerable amount of 'custom and practice' amongst a work group that was accepted by previous managers.

If, as a nurse manager, you find some of these points applicable, it is still necessary to take as constructive a view as possible of your own part in industrial relations management. This will be achieved if you adopt an appropriate attitude to problems of managing conflict, if you improve your knowledge of matters relevant to dealing with trade unions and employee relations' problems, as well as acquiring the personal skills needed to manage such problems.

CONFLICT AND INDUSTRIAL RELATIONS

We discussed in Chapter 15 the general topic of conflict as a feature of organisational life and the various means by which senior nurses could manage this for constructive purposes. In the particular circumstances of the relationship between 'employees' and 'employers' it should be recognised that there are some conflicts of interest as well as a range of common interests. Managers have to accept that there is no unrestricted 'right to manage', that employees have a right to consider their own interests in work as well as responsibilities towards their employer and that some agreed balance has to be achieved. In coming to terms with this fact of industrial relations management, it can be useful to analyse the sources of potential conflict between employees and employers.

Employees' objectives

Most people look for satisfaction of several requirements through their work; broadly this will include some of the following:

— Satisfactory pay and security of income
— Security of employment
— Job satisfaction

— Satisfactory conditions (hours, holidays, sick pay etc.)
— Satisfactory working environment (clean, safe, good facilities etc.)
— Satisfactory social environment (friendly work group, personal contacts)
— Prospects for advancement
— Satisfactory seniors/supervisor.

The priorities which individuals identify will vary. Some look for the highest earnings while for others job satisfaction is more important.

Employers' objectives

Broadly the owners or shareholders in a commercial enterprise will be seeking satisfaction of one or more of the following aims:

— Satisfactory return on the capital invested (not just 'profit' but a specific rate of earnings or growth)
— Security of investment and business continuation
— Future growth of the business
— Prestige and privilege from ownership
— Power from ownership
— Social satisfaction (interest in particular products, services, providing employment, contribution to community etc.).

As with employees, priorities will vary with different individuals and in different business cultures.

In the 'health care business' the objectives of 'employers' will seem to be different from those of overtly commercial companies. The ultimate purpose of the NHS is to make health care available to all communities using the financial provisions made available by the government of the day. Thus as an employer the aims are providing community services in the most cost-effective manner. In the private health care sector there is a similar aim of providing services, but to individual customers or clients at a price that will enable the organisation to survive, and, in some cases, make a trading profit.

When employee and employer objectives are set down side by side it can be seen that they are not automatically compatible. If employees seek increases in pay, this will increase the costs of a service unless something else is done to prevent this. Health authorities seeking to modify the methods of delivering care or trying to improve efficiency will introduce new processes and methods of working. Although it can be argued that such improvements are in the long-term interest of staff as well, there will be clashes of interest with those who fear changes in their job content, earnings or status.

The essential aim in industrial relations management is to achieve a pragmatic balance between the need for organisational efficiency and the need for employee satisfaction. Although this purpose is applicable to all work-places as a response to the inherent conflict, it is evident that in some it is harder to achieve. Some industries and organisations are more 'conflict and dispute prone' than others. There are many causes, such as size of the work force, concentration in large units, geographical location, history of labour relations, degree of centralisation and management personnel policies; but two of the most significant are likely to be the work systems and the method of payment.

Work systems

The 'technology' used to provide services or manufacture products has a major influence on the nature of employee jobs, social interactions and methods of supervision. Some systems involve staff in work tasks that have little intrinsic satisfaction, and place them under constant pressure with close but unsupportive supervision. Within a hospital it is possible to identify contrasting 'production technologies' and consequent demands on staff (intensive care units, hospital laundry, accident department, patient records' office etc.). It is to be expected that there will be potentially greater conflict between staff and management, as well as between staff themselves, in some of these units than in others.

Payment systems

The amount of pay taken home by staff can be a source of dissatisfaction if they consider it to be less than their worth. This feeling can emerge from comparisons with other workers, both inside the organisation and outside. It is inevitable that there will be differences in rates of remuneration for different occupations. But the aim of management should not be to pay the least to everyone unless forced to pay more, but to create a pay structure that is seen to be fair by staff as a reasonable reflection of differing skills, responsibilities and scarcity. This aim has to be balanced against the need to control and minimise labour costs. The use of incentive schemes or merit payments can increase staff earnings but can also be a source of disagreement on grounds of equity. Similarly, excessive use of overtime and special pay allowances can be a source of argument as can the frequent employment of temporary or contract staff at higher pay rates than permanent employees. There is no easy answer to problems of maintaining a pay system that is fair to all employees and the requirements of the employing authority, but there are trends towards simpler pay structures and the use of 'job evaluation' techniques. We have included a brief account of the main forms of job evaluation.

Job evaluation

The overall purpose of an evaluation exercise is to make an objective comparison of the content of a number of jobs in the same organisation. It is not intended as a means of assessing individual competence. The outcome should be to allocate pay differentials in a way that reflects the differences in job content. In practice, evaluation schemes are not objective, as the judgment about the comparative worth of different jobs is still made by individuals or committees. This involves subjective opinions and some negotiation. The intention, however, is to make this process as dispassionate as possible.

For all the various methods of job evaluation it is important to start with reliable job descriptions. From this base there are three common ways of making comparisons.

Ranking

In this approach the jobs to be evaluated are placed in order of difficulty and contribution. When the order has been agreed between the evaluators this can be converted into a simple grading where jobs are placed together into a few categories which are to receive the same rate of pay. If eight jobs are to be evaluated (A,B,C,D,E,F,G,H) and are judged to be ranked as C,E,F,A,G,B,H and D, the final decision may be to place these into four distinct pay grades, jobs C and E in grade one, F, A and G in grade two, B and H in grade three and D in grade four.

Classification

This relatively simple method starts with the definition of grading criteria, and then, based on assessments of particular jobs, allocates them to the most appropriate grade. Typically five to seven different grades are identified.

Grade A Simple tasks under close supervision
Grade B Tasks requiring the knowledge of a limited number of clearly set out tasks, simple operations requiring manual dexterity, low level of responsibility, work checked and inspected
Grade C Routine work more responsible than B, checking grade B work
Grade D Some initiative required, routine will alter, little supervision given
Grade E Special knowledge required, individual responsibility, control over sequence of work, or over small groups of people
Grade F Supervision of sections, responsible for complete divisions of work, contact management regularly, needs special experience, discretion, judgement or knowledge.

Points rating

This is a more detailed approach in which jobs are compared by some common elements: these may be (i) mental requirements, (ii) skill content, (iii) physical effort and (iv) working conditions. There can be more complex factors in this approach. Each element is allocated a range of possible points so that individual jobs can be awarded the appropriate number to reflect the comparative skill difference or physical difficulty etc. There may not be an equal allocation to each sub-category. Weighting is usually in favour of the 'mental' and 'skill' elements. These may have a range 0 to 40 points each, whilst 'physical effort' and 'working conditions' may have 0 to 20.

The total points allocation for each job can then be plotted on a 'scatter graph' to examine how far the existing pay structure varies from the one suggested by job evaluation. A mean, or adjusted mean, can be calculated and pay steps or grades for the preferred structure created (see Fig. 21.1). Jobs below the mean can be given pay increases either immediately or in stages to bring them into line. Jobs considered to be overpaid in the existing arrangement will be gradually adjusted.

These descriptions of job evaluations are rather simplified to give an overall appreciation of how they are intended to work. In practice there will be considerable industrial relations repercussions and protracted negotiations involved in modifying a pay structure.

Merit payments

There seems to be an attractive logic in a pay policy which pays staff, who show greater effort and responsibility than their colleagues doing the same job, higher rewards. The system of 'merit pay' attempts to achieve this. There are, however, several criticisms of such an approach — the most significant being doubt on whether it is possible to make fair differentiation between individuals and whether the likely animosity will reduce the value of such a policy. The policy can be used to set up a 'wage drift' where there is a gradual increase in pay as everyone is awarded a merit increase.

In an attempt to control merit pay some organisations adopt a system with a similar format to that of performance review and appraisal (see Ch. 20), where individuals are compared on a number of specific factors in carrying out their job tasks. 'Quantity', 'quality', 'effort', 'relationships', 'attendance', 'punctuality', etc. are common aspects. Individuals who are rated higher than average on these elements can be awarded specific merit increases, or given a higher than average increase at the annual pay review.

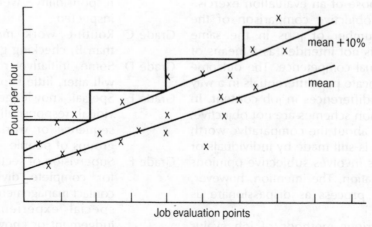

Fig. 21.1 Scatter diagram.

Incentive schemes

In manufacturing industry there has been a tradition of 'payment by results' for employees working on production tasks. The simplest form is 'piecework' where individuals are paid an agreed sum for each item produced. More common are schemes of payment based on a 'bonus' or 'incentive' payment above basic pay, in return for output higher than the minimum or standard performance. There is a need to establish accurately a definition of standard performance and this involves the techniques of 'work measurement'.

There are several commonly used methods of establishing the base for incentive payment. The application of a stop watch to allocate set times to the component parts of a task is probably the most common. In the 'time study', a work study engineer selects appropriate elements to measure but in doing so also assesses whether an individual is working at a 'standard rate'; this is regarded as the rate at which a qualified worker who was motivated to apply himself to work would perform; this may be compared to walking at four miles an hour or dealing a pack of cards into four trays in thirty seconds.

From each observation of a job cycle the time study engineer records the time taken and the observed rating. These figures are converted into 'basic time' by the formula:

$$\frac{\text{Observed time} \times \text{Observed rating}}{\text{Standard rate}} = \text{Basic time}$$

If an activity was measured to take 0.24 minutes with the employee working at 95 standard (less than standard) the calculation would be:

$$\frac{0.24 \text{ mins} \times 95}{100} = 0.228 \text{ mins}$$

When all the elements have been calculated it is necessary to decide on the work standard, depending on policy, ease of identification, the costing etc. to be taken into account in producing a calculated standard time. This is further modified by the addition of allowances for rest and fatigue (range from 8% to 20%);

above this, further allowances may be made for contingency or other factors. Finally a standard time can be agreed.

There are other ways of assessing the standard times for work. One is the use of 'synthetics'. This requires the reference to data from previous time studies to find common elements with other jobs to be measured. Where these are present it is possible to calculate a standard time once a method of working is agreed. This can be useful in estimating the cost involved in new work or in comparing likely gains from a change in method. Another work measurement technique is known as 'predetermined motion time systems' (PMTS) which relies on assessments that have been made of work in industrial environments identified as common smaller elements. This data can be used to allocate such standard times to the components of a particular cycle of work. In another technique, 'analytical estimating', a person qualified in a particular task is asked to estimate the time needed. This is used where work is non-repetitive or more highly skilled, making time study difficult. Another approach is that of 'activity sampling'. Here an observer makes a series of instantaneous random observations of a number of workers performing a task. Such data can be built up to make a complete picture of a particular task, although several calculations have to be made to take account of the likely errors in sampling and bias.

Where work measurement information is to be used to form the basis of an incentive scheme, further calculations are required. The standard hours or minutes taken from the study can be compared with the time actually taken by a worker. Where the time taken is the same as standard time this is regarded as a '100 performance'. It is then common to commence bonus payments from a 75 performance with progressive steps to 100 where a 33.3% bonus could be earned and then pro rata payment beyond 100. This formula may be varied with different circumstances and different employers. It is unlikely that staff will be able to work continuously against standard time throughout a shift. Many schemes will therefore include compensations for 'waiting time', 'unmeasured work' etc. This will be included in the final calculation of bonus payment.

This system of payment was pioneered in manufacturing environments but has been extended into service and public sector organisations. Within the health service there have been incentive schemes introduced for ancillary and maintenance staff. There is considerable controversy about the merits of incentive. In practice it is difficult to establish acceptable standards and to ensure that there is a fair link between effort and reward. There have been examples where schemes have got out of control and been withdrawn by management, or have been the subject of disputes with the work force. There are usually increases in output when schemes are first introduced, but there are also increases in administration costs and minor disputes over the fairness of times and the accuracy of bonus calculations.

As a result of these unattractive features there has been a move towards developing pay systems which encourage high productivity but have more simplicity and acceptability. The use of 'measured day work' is one of the common systems to replace incentive payment. Here, specific standards are agreed for particular jobs and a rate of pay attached to each. An individual will be expected to maintain an average performance as agreed with her supervisor. This forms the basis of a contract where management agrees to maintain the supply of work and the operative agrees to maintain the level of work. These agreements can be changed by individuals who are able to work at a higher rate or wish to drop to a lower one.

Most nurse managers will find such methods of payment are not relevant to the tasks involved in nursing. In their inter-face with other parts of a health care work force and in contributing to the general management of a unit it can be necessary to develop an understanding of incentive or measured day work schemes that are in operation in a health care organisation.

Other areas of knowledge that may be needed by nurse managers in contributing to the effective management of industrial relations will include an understanding of trade union organisation, an appreciation of employment legislation and the application of negotiation skills (see Ch. 11), grievance handling skills (see Ch. 16) and discipline handling skills (see Ch. 17). Over and above these general management considerations it is necessary for senior nurses to have an understanding of the specific industrial relations agreements, procedures, policies and 'customs and practices' in their particular organisations.

TRADE UNIONS

Structures of unions

A trade union can be defined in general terms as: 'A continuous association of wage earners for the purpose of maintaining and improving the condition of their working lives'.

Trade unions did not develop for the benefit of society as a whole. They were created from a necessity for working people to have greater power in the relationship with their employers than they could establish as individuals. Trade unions still place the interests of their own members first. The overall aims of the trade union movement have been summarised by the Trades Union Congress (TUC) as:

1. Improved terms of employment
2. Improved physical environment at work
3. Full employment and national prosperity
4. Security of income and employment
5. Improved social security
6. Fair shares in national income and wealth
7. Industrial democracy
8. A voice in government
9. Improved public and social services
10. Public control and planning of industry.

In 1986 there were some 12 million trade union members in the UK, from a working population of 26 million. The proportion and number of trade union members remained relatively static over twenty years, although there has been a decline in total numbers in some unions reflecting changes in employment patterns during the mid 1980s.

There are some 450 separate trade unions, each with its own constitution and separate sphere of influence. There are differences in size, type of worker represented, industries covered and historical development. This makes general statements about trade unions difficult to substantiate. Many unions are small and specialised. Those with significant membership number less than 100 with the most influential being fewer still. Thus 90% of all trade union members are found in the top 40 unions with over 50 000 members each. Despite the variety it is possible to find some basic, common elements in their organisation.

In origin all unions are democratic institutions. There is a continual need to ensure that the rank and file members have an influence in the activities of a union as there is a tendency for full-time officers of any voluntary organisation to have the monopoly of power. The means to control this excess are the constitution and rules which should provide the framework for ordinary members to determine policy.

In the trade union movement the basic unit of organisation — the branch — is intended as the link with rank and file members. On joining a union an individual becomes a member of one branch which in most cases is based on a geographical area covering several employing organisations. This can cause problems as most members are concerned with the affairs related to their employer; thus attendance at local branch meetings may be low. Now many unions are developing more work-place meetings. In the case of major NHS unions there will be meetings at particular hospitals for members.

The importance of the work-place organisation has been reinforced by the increased influence of local shop stewards. They normally carry out union tasks on a part-time, voluntary basis and are therefore 'lay' officials of a union.

At branch level members will elect a committee to carry on its affairs. The branch secretary is usually the most significant appointment, together with the chairman and treasurer. Most unions have part-time lay officers in these posts, although some employers will grant time and in some large unions the secretary is a full-time salaried post.

The next unit of organisation above the branch is the district, region or division. Committees here are mostly made up of delegates from branch committees and again are likely to be lay officers. The committee at branch or district level is able to appoint full-time organisers; this is most common for districts. The national policy and major business of trade unions is in the hands of a national executive committee or council. The size and method of appointment varies with different unions. The executive of the General and Municipal Workers Union is formed by nominations from each of its ten regions plus two members from the regional council and the full-time officer. The National Association of Local Government Officers describes its structure in its handbook as:

Every member belongs to a branch, composed solely of fellow employees in his own service. Branches send delegates to the Association's annual conference, where policy is decided. The policy is carried out by a National Executive Council (the NEC) which is elected each year by a ballot of all members. In addition, branches send delegates to a district council — the main link between members, branches and the NEC.

At the national level the key post is generally that of general secretary or, in some cases, the president. The process of appointment to the top post varies from being selected by the national executive from amongst its number, to election by the total membership, the individual then holding the post until retirement. An issue in organisation for the large general unions is the need to have some means of representing the interests of different work groups. Thus there may be a 'trade group' structure (Transport and General Workers Union) or separate structures for major sections (National Association of Local Government Officers). The main check on policy by lay members is through the 'delegate conferences'. These vary in size and structure but for the large unions are likely to be annual affairs with 500 attending, bringing proposals from branches which will be debated with other motions from district and national level.

Full-time officials attend the conference and are able to speak on motions but are not generally given the right to vote. Thus the conference should provide policy guidelines and endorsement for the actions of the NEC; but full-time national officers will wish to influence decisions, not just wait passively for directives. Throughout trade union history there have been several conflicting factors that have influenced the direction of development. There has been a trend towards amalgamation of small unions to reflect changes in employment patterns, but the advantages have to be set against the need to protect the minority interests. There is a need to provide professional services and efficient administration which has to be balanced against the need for democracy and accountability. Current trends suggest that unions will continue to amalgamate. There is likely to be better administration and more sophisticated means of communicating with members. At local level the shop steward is likely to remain the predominant influence, but is likely to be better trained and supported.

Shop stewards

For some managers the prospect of having to deal with a shop steward fills them with alarm. This reaction is the result of a stereotyped view that all work-place representatives are militants who are determined to make life as difficult as possible for managers. Such attitudes amongst managers are bound to harm the industrial relations climate in their organisation, and are based on ignorance.

It is estimated that there are some 250 000 shop stewards in this country representing manual and non-manual workers. Their political views as well as their personality characteristics and levels of competency spread across the spectrum. Managers have to come to terms with the fact that stewards are here to stay and should endeavour to build as constructive relationships as possible. This requires an understanding of their role and their problems.

All stewards do the job on a voluntary basis with 95% doing so in addition to their full-time employment. Under the guidelines in the ACAS Code of Practice shop stewards should be given the right to reasonable time and facilities during working hours to attend to union business. However, the actual interpretation of this is subject to negotiation with management.

A steward will represent a specific group of staff ranging from a handful to a hundred. His time will be spent on administrative tasks (checking membership, passing circulars etc.), on liaison tasks (talking with members, consulting with management etc.) and negotiation tasks (progressing grievances, seeking improvements in conditions etc.). The communication and liaison activities generally take most time, but stewards regard negotiation with management as their most important, and difficult task.

Authority is derived from several sources. Where an employer has made a recognition agreement with a union it is likely that this will contain rights and powers for work-place representatives, as will the grievance and disciplinary procedures. The fact that a work group have selected a representative adds to his legitimacy, as do credentials from his union, and support from branch or district officers. In recent years there has been acceptance of the rights of shop stewards by the Employment Act and the Health and Safety at Work Act.

There will be differences in the way that individual representatives approach their role. Some seek to be leaders, influencing the attitude and actions of their members. Others see themselves as following the wishes of their group, and will be unwilling to enter into commitments with management without continual reference back. The problem for most stewards is that they can be at the

---

**WORK PLACE REPRESENTATIVES'
ACTIVITIES**

Collect Union subscription
Check Union membership cards
Stop members falling into arrears with dues
Arrange regular meetings with members to keep
  them informed
Attend regular meetings with management to keep
  informed
Arrange regular meetings with other trade union
  representatives
Arrange special meetings with members
Attend special meetings with management
Attend special meetings with other representatives
Prepare and present group cases and individual cases
  to management
Negotiate with management (local, senior and
  personnel)
Circulate members to keep informed
Advance Union membership by recruiting new
  members
Introduce new members to work customs and
  practices
Ensure apprentice training carried out
Seek information from management
Attend Safety committees
Advise members on Safety regulations
Check conditions and facilities to ensure safe and
  healthy working
Advise members of procedures to claim protection
  etc.
Ensure members abide by Safety rules
Report accident details to Branch
Attend Branch meetings
Keep notice board up to date with Branch and
  National Information
Encourage members to attend Branch meetings
Use Branch services as required
Use Area/National services as required
Send written reports to Branch and District officials
Ensure members keep to rules for own benefit
Ensure members keep to agreements
Ensure members keep to existing customs and
  practices
Keep in touch with members' problems, views etc.
Monitor overtime working

Fig. 21.2 The tasks of work place representatives.

crunch point between the interests of their section, local management objectives, union policies and the politics of the local shop steward network. In trying to do their best some will lose the support of their workmates and others will be seen as disruptive influences by local managers. It is not surprising to find a high turnover amongst stewards.

In most procedures shop stewards find they are required to meet local and junior managers in trying to resolve problems. Stewards tend to be dismissive of the quality of managers at this level, finding them poorly informed and reluctant to deal with issues themselves.

Nurse managers have an increasing involvement with representatives of the unions representing nursing staff as well as ancillary workers. There has been an increased militancy in many health service shop stewards during the 1980s, partly caused by resource and pay shortages, but probably accentuated by procrastinating and negative local management. Nurse managers should be willing and sufficiently competent to try to cultivate constructive relations at this level by proper consultation and a recognition of the rights and problems of representatives.

Trades Union Congress

In this description of trade unions we have been concerned with differences and similarities between individual unions. For over 100 years there has been a recognition within the movement of the need for co-operation between unions. The main framework for this is the TUC (Trades Union Congress). This is like a club to which trade unions can become affiliated members. There is an annual meeting with delegates from affiliated unions — this is the actual Congress — and a number of full-time officers and a range of committees to carry out Congress policy and provide advisory services to member unions. The most influential post is that of General Secretary (Norman Willis). There are 88 affiliated trade unions in the TUC (1986) with 9.5 million members.

Trade unions in the NHS

There are a large number of trade unions with health care workers in the membership. There are several with nursing memberships which have been granted recognition (right to bargain and represent members at local and national level):

— *Confederation of Health Service Employees (COHSE)*. Caters for all grades of staff within the Health Service and claims the largest number of nurses amongst its membership.
— *General and Municipal Workers Union (GMWU)*. One of the largest general unions but with a relatively small number of nursing members who belong to the administrative section MATSA (Managerial Administrative, Technical and Supervisory Association)
— *National Association of Local Government Officers (NALGO)*. A large 'white collar' union with significant nurse membership. There is a Health Service section with a National Officer dealing specifically with the Service.
— *National Union of Public Employees (NUPE)*. A large union with members throughout the public sector. There are a large number of nurse members, particularly from the auxiliary grades.
— *Transport and General Workers Union (TGWU)*. The largest general union in the UK, but with only a relatively small number of nurse members.

All these trade unions are registered with the Certification Officer under the terms of the Trade Union and Labour Relations Act, and thus are registered independent unions. They are all affiliated to the TUC.

There are a number of other organisations with bargaining rights in the NHS representing nurses, but in origin they are more professional institutions than trade unions. Although these are all now registered, some remain outside the TUC.

— *Health Visitors Association (HVA)*. A small organisation for health visitors and school nurses (associate grade members), it is TUC affiliated. The Scottish Health Visitors Association has a similar function.
— *Royal College of Midwives (RCM)*. An organisation of midwives and pupil midwives with an educational as well as a trade union function.
— *Royal College of Nursing of the United Kingdom (RCN)*. An organisation for nurses holding a statutory qualification, or those training for a qualification, which acts as a professional and educational body as well as a trade union.

COLLECTIVE BARGAINING IN THE NHS

Terms and conditions of employment in the Health Service are established centrally so that there is a national salary structure and other national conditions which local health authorities are obliged to meet. There are also a number of 'procedural agreements', establishing rights for employees and the appropriate way to deal with such problems as discipline, grievance, redundancies and unit closures.

The activities which precede the annual 'substantive' agreements are partly contained in negotiations within the Whitley Council framework and partly through the Pay Review Body. In 1986 there were ten Whitley Councils empowered to negotiate on terms of employment for NHS staff: administrative and clerical; ambulancemen; ancillary staffs; medical and (hospital) dental; nurses and midwives; optical staffs; pharmaceutical staffs; professional and technical staffs (A and B), dental (local authorities).

Until 1983 nurses' pay was established by the appropriate councils. Since then a Pay Review Body, with an independent chairman and seven members from outside the Health Service, hears evidence from trade unions, DHSS and other interested parties concerning the proper amount of pay awards. The body reports directly to the government recommending a salary level which it may, or may not, accept.

The special Whitley Councils continue to review other aspects of nurses' conditions. In addition there is the General Whitley Council for the Health Service which sets conditions that have general application (removal expenses, redundancy payments etc.). Nurse managers need to be familiar with the content of handbooks issued by the Nurses' and

Midwives' Whitley Council and the General Council as these contain useful information on conditions and procedures.

The national structures which establish this Service-wide structure of salaries and conditions have been supplemented at local level by a number of Joint Consultative Committees. The intention of this arrangement has been to promote 'the closest co-operation and provide a recognised means of consultation between health authorities, its senior officers and staff' (Whitley Council Handbook). Within the Service, as in industry generally, there are different experiences in how effective such formal joint consultation can be. Most nurse managers will be involved at the even more local and less formal end of collective bargaining and consultation in that they may be members of committees and working parties, as well as meeting with shop stewards to deal with matters concerning local work practices, working conditions, staff discipline and staff complaints.

Thus it is essential that they acquire an understanding of the role and problems of shop floor representatives and their place in trade union organisation.

CONSULTATION AND NEGOTIATION

The ability to consult with others (exchange views on matters of mutual interest or to seek information as a preliminary to decision-making) and to negotiate with others (seek to reach agreement on issues involving conflict) is an important aspect of general management that is relevant to nurse managers. We have included a discussion of this topic in Chapter 11, but there are a few additional considerations in applying this to an industrial relations context.

Senior nurses are unlikely to be greatly involved in negotiating changes in pay or conditions of service but are expected to play a part in the introduction of new working practices and to resolve local disagreements with staff. Problem-solving at any level in industrial relations demands obtaining infor-

mation to develop understanding, clarifying aims and planning positive means to resolve conflicts as a preliminary to action.

Consultation meetings with staff and shop stewards can provide valuable information and form the basis for constructive solutions. Trade union representatives complain, however, that meetings convened by managers as consultative often turn out to be attempts by them to impose changes or decisions that have already been formulated. Assuming a genuine desire by managers to find common interest and reach mutual understanding, there are a number of questions to be considered:

1. For what reasons do management or staff want to change the 'status quo'?
2. What changes are likely to be acceptable and practical for management and staff?
3. What are the underlying causes of staff complaints or resistance to proposals?
4. What are the points of common interest/agreement between managers, trade union representatives and staff?
5. Are representatives really representing their members' wishes and views?
6. Who has the most power and influence in the situation?

Consultation meetings can be convened separately or form the preliminary stage of a meeting that continues as a negotiation or decision-making session.

In negotiation it is essential to prepare before each meeting; this will enable managers to think through a number of important issues:

1. What do we hope to achieve at this meeting?
2 Is this really a consultation or negotiation meeting?
3. Who should attend?
4. What information should we prepare?
5. What information should be given out before the meeting and to whom should it be given?
6. What are the main points of our 'case'?
7. What are likely to be the main points of their 'case'?

8. What ideally do we want as an agreement?
9. What is the minimum acceptable to us?
10. What are they likely to want as an ideal agreement?
11. What is the minimum they are likely to accept?
12. What will we do if deadlock is reached?
13. Who should lead the negotiation?
14. Who will take notes for us?
15. What is the proposed agenda?
16. What authority do we have to reach agreement?
17. How much authority do trade union representatives have to reach agreement?
18. What arrangements should be made to report back progress or the outcome of the meeting to staff?
19. Have we got the support of more senior management for our aims?
20. What time-scale are we working to in resolving this issue?

Managers should try to conduct all meetings in a constructive and orderly manner, but when negotiating there are three main choices of overall strategy. In the first, management negotiators would make a direct statement of their requirements to settle a dispute and press trade union representatives to accept this as practical and reasonable. The second is for managers to seek an understanding of trade union requirements or position in the matter without declaring management position or views. The third possibility is for management to overstate its demands, or understate any offers, as an opening gambit in the bargaining process. This approach is generally employed in wage negotiations or other matters where a compromise will have to be arranged. The second strategy is most constructive in local negotiations as it enables management to start with an understanding of the trade union's most extreme position, which might be acceptable to management. If not, management might still be able to put together some acceptable compromise. The first approach allows no room for manoeuvre, thus is most likely to lead to deadlock. With proper preparation of facts and broad

strategy, management will be better able to control each negotiating meeting. One model which can be used to run meetings is:

1. Clarify purpose and management authority in an opening statement by senior manager present.
2. A brief outline of the problem background and summary of any previous meetings by management spokesman.
3. An 'agenda' for the meeting suggested by management spokesman for acceptance by trade union side.
4. Management seeks a statement from staff representatives of their views, demands or offers (if following strategy two).
5. Management questions trade union statements to gain full understanding but without commitment.
6. Management rejects parts of union 'case' that are unacceptable but puts counter-suggestions as constructively as possible.
7. Management tries to encourage discussion of their 'offer' and to prevent instant rejection.
8. If deadlock seems likely or further information is needed, management suggests adjournment.
9. After adjournment, management summarises position and seeks further compromise from union negotiators or makes fresh offer as appropriate.
10. Process continues until meeting concluded. Management summarises areas of agreement and disagreement. Care should be taken to ensure that details of any agreement are really understood and agreed by both 'sides'.
11. Next step agreed — implementation of agreement or further meetings, or conciliation/arbitration by third party, or refer to next stage of disputes procedure, or unilateral action threatened by either party.
12. Agree who and how to communicate the outcome of the meeting to staff not present.
13. Write notes, minutes or detailed agreement. Refer to senior manager or IR

specialist if appropriate. In many cases shop stewards will wish to refer issues or management offers back to their members for their acceptance. Management should try to establish whether the shop stewards will be recommending acceptance or not.

Although most senior nurses will not be involved in substantial negotiations with trade union representatives until they progress into the ranks of general management it is still important to be properly informed and skilled in handling aspects of labour relations. During the 1970s and 80s there has been an increase in legislation by various governments which has a direct bearing on the relationship between employees and employers. This is also an area where all managers require at least a general appreciation.

EMPLOYMENT LEGISLATION

Employment protection

Individual employees have a number of rights in relation to their employment. Several are contained in the Employment Protection (Consolidation) Act 1978. This Act consolidates earlier legislation (Redundancy Payment Act 1965, Contract of Employment Act 1972, Trade Union and Labour Relations Act 1974 and 1976, Employment Protection Act 1975), and was itself modified by the Employment Acts of 1980 and 1982.

One important part of this legislation which nurses should understand is the rights employees have not to be unfairly dismissed from their employment. In the event of dismissal it is possible to complain to an industrial tribunal. In addition to protection in the obvious circumstances where an employee is sacked, the protection against unfair dismissal can also apply to fixed-term contracts, refusal to reinstate after absence for pregnancy and where employees resign due to action by the employer (constructive dismissal). The underlying principles of their protection should not prevent employers dismissing unsatisfactory employees, but it requires them

to have a valid reason and to act reasonably in treating that reason as fair. A valid reason for dismissal should fall within one of five categories:

1. Conduct: Dismissal due to misconduct on the part of an employee
2. Capacity: Dismissal due to employee's inability, or lack of qualification to do a satisfactory job
3. Redundancy: Dismissal as employer has no work, or insufficient work for employee
4. A statutory requirement: Loss of qualification to perform necessary duties.
5. Some other substantial reason: Most reasons are contained under the above headings, but it is possible for an employer to seek justification of dismissal as fair for some other reason.

It is unfair to dismiss employees for joining or participating in trade union activities at an appropriate time. Similarly, it is unfair to dismiss an employee for refusing to join a trade union, except in some special trade union membership (closed shop) agreements. It is unfair to dismiss an employee simply on the grounds of pregnancy. There are further stipulations about dismissal during industrial action which broadly give employers the right to dismiss all who take part in the action, but if selected individuals are dismissed they have a right to refer this to the industrial tribunal.

It is important for line managers in nursing, as for managers everywhere, to be aware of further protection given to employees (and therefore themselves as individual employers) for dismissal procedures to be seen to be fair. The reasons for dismissal should be explained clearly and procedures followed that are consistent with the ACAS (Advisory, Conciliation and Arbitration Service) code of conduct.

Large employers are expected to conform closely to the code and to keep satisfactory written records of disciplinary cases.

The principles that should underlie disciplinary procedures are firstly that employees should know what standards of conduct are expected of them. Rules should be readily available and explained to employees; it is recommended that employees are given copies of the main rules concerning safe and efficient working conditions and for the maintenance of satisfactory relationships.

There are eleven features that should be present in a satisfactory procedure:

1. Should be in writing.
2. Specify to whom it should apply.
3. Provide for matters to be dealt with quickly.
4. Indicate the disciplinary actions which may be taken.
5. Specify levels of management which have authority to take the various forms of disciplinary action.
6. Provide for individuals to be informed of the complaints against them and have the opportunity to state their case before decisions are reached.
7. Give individuals the right to be accompanied by a trade union representative or a fellow employee of their choice.
8. Ensure that, except for gross misconduct, no employee is dismissed for a first breach of discipline.
9. Ensure that disciplinary action is not taken before careful investigation.
10. Ensure individuals are given an explanation for any penalties imposed.
11. Provide a right of appeal and specify the procedures to follow.

All employees can complain against a dismissal if: (i) they work for at least 16 hours a week, (ii) have worked continuously for one year (if less than 20 employees this is extended to 2 years), (iii) they work at least eight hours a week and have been in continuous employment for five years. Thus individuals who are normally excluded from the right

include: freelancers and independent contractors; those over normal retiring age; fixed term contracts where an individual previously agrees in writing to forego rights of complaint.

There are several other aspects of employment protection which can be relevant to health care managers, notably: constructive dismissal; dismissal associated with maternity; dismissal in connection with criminal offences; dismissal connected with illness; dismissal on grounds of redundancy. It is outside the scope of this book to provide detail on all these points. Nurse managers should be generally aware of their existence but be particularly knowledgeable about the disciplinary rules and standards of their own unit, about their health authority procedure and about their own authority in disciplinary matters. There is a belief amongst some senior nurses that it is no longer possible to dismiss unsatisfactory employees. This is certainly not the case. It is essential for line managers to be properly informed, to act in a professional manner and to seek appropriate advice when they are confronted with this problem.

Sex discrimination

The Sex Discrimination Act (1975) makes sex discrimination against women unlawful in employment, training and related matters. Individuals have a right of direct access to the civil courts and industrial tribunals for legal remedies for unlawful discrimination. The Equal Opportunities Commission is the main source of advice about this Act and the Equal Pay Act (1970).

This Act is a complex piece of legislation but it is necessary for line managers in health care to be aware of the general principles involved and then to seek more expert advice on the particular applications in their place of employment.

The Act identifies 'direct sex discrimination' where a woman is treated less favourably than a man on the grounds of her sex, and 'indirect sex discrimination' as treatment which may be described as equal in a formal sense but discriminatory in its effect on one sex. There are similar unlawful discriminations against married persons.

Discrimination may be evident in the policy and practice of recruitment or in opportunities for promotion, training, benefits and facilities. There are exceptions to these general rules in that an employer may offer special treatment to women in connection with pregnancy or childbirth without unlawfully discriminating.

The main exceptions are concerned with 'genuine occupational qualifications'. Here employers are required to demonstrate that in providing opportunities for promotion or transfer or training, or in recruiting staff for a particular job, the preference for one sex over the other is a genuine requirement of the job. The likely reasons are physiological, decency or privacy, living-in requirements, single sex establishments, providing personal welfare services, legal restrictions, work outside the UK and employing married couples. There are also a number of 'special employment cases' of which midwifery is one. Under the Act the legal restrictions for men becoming midwives are removed, but it is not unlawful for employers to discriminate in selecting or training midwives.

Health and safety at work

As the purpose of all health care organisations is to care for the sick and to promote good health it would seem reasonable for health care workers to expect that everything possible would be done to protect their own health and safety whilst at work. This expectation has been reinforced by the Health and Safety at Work Act (1974) whereby certain obligations are placed on employers to provide safe and healthy environments.

The application of the Act has been difficult within the NHS for several reasons: the size of the organisation, the wide variety of potential health and safety hazards, the management structure and the application of 'crown immunity' to NHS premises, are some of the most significant.

Despite these problems it is essential for senior nurses to appreciate the general concepts contained in this legislation as well as the particular regulations and procedures that apply to their units. Some of the significant general principles are:

It shall be the duty of every employer to ensure, as far as is reasonably practicable, the health, safety and welfare at work of all his employees.
(Section 247)

This generally applies in particular to:

the provision and maintenance of plant and systems of work that are, so far as is reasonably practicable, safe and without risks to health.
(Section 2,2(a))

Similar provisions apply to 'use, handling, storage and transport of articles and substances', which covers everything used at work and all work activities. Other requirements cover the provision of instruction, training and supervision; the maintenance of work places and means of entry and exit; the adequacy of facilities and arrangements for welfare, and the need to provide a written statement of safety policy for the attention of all employees. There is a requirement to have employee safety representatives and safety committees.

Under the Act there are obligations also to protect the health and safety of members of the public, as well as the employees of subcontractors etc. who work on an employer's premises. The terms of the Act are extremely broad in an attempt to cover most people and most circumstances.

There are further extensive responsibilities for manufacturers, suppliers and installers of plant, equipment, substances, etc., to ensure that their products are designed and installed safely.

Throughout the Act the words 'as far as is reasonably practical' appear. This indicates the difficulty in prescribing exactly the standard of acceptable risk to health and safety. There are three sources of more detailed standards. The Health and Safety at Work Act did not replace existing legislation, so that a number of Acts exist giving more detailed standards such as the Factories Act, Office,

Shop and Railway Premises Act, and the Shop Act. In addition, there are a large number of Safety Regulations which give more precise specifications on particular health hazards (asbestos, lead, etc.), machinery hazards and on particular industries. A third source of guidance are the various Codes of Practice. Although not having the force of law they can be used by health and safety inspectors to persuade employers.

The Act also places obligations on all individual employees to co-operate with an employer to carry out his duties, to take 'reasonable care for the health and safety of himself and other persons' and not to 'intentionally or recklessly interfere with or misuse anything provided in the interests of health, safety or welfare' (Section 7).

There are three main systems of compulsion on an employer to provide and maintain a safe and healthy place of work — improvement notices, prohibition notices and fines or threats of imprisonment. The health and safety executive inspectors have the power to inspect premises and issue notices. The executive is also a source of advice and infor-mation which can refer to the employment medical advisory service. The issue of protecting staff from health and safety hazards within a hospital or other health care establishment is a major problem. There has been concern and some criticism of health authorities on failures to protect patients adequately. Similarly, criticism of health authority practice towards staff has been evident. Ward level nurse managers have a clear responsibility to encourage staff to maintain the highest standards and practices in their own work areas and to make representations to higher management where the environment is unsatisfactory.

REFERENCES

Brewster C 1985 Understanding industrial relations. Pan, London
Industrial relations handbook 1980 HMSO, London
Kinnersley P 1974 The hazards of work. Pluto Press, London
Lewis D 1986 Essentials of employment law. IPM, Wimbledon
Thomson G 1984 A textbook of industrial relations management. IPM, Wimbledon

Financing the NHS

Health Service accounting

Cost accounting

Budgetary control

Nurse managers and finance

22
Financial management

All nurse managers should have an understanding of at least four basic aspects of finance related to health care. They should appreciate where the money that is used to provide patient services and to run their organisations comes from, they should understand how costs for different parts of the service can be assessed; they should appreciate how the system of budgetary control works; and it will also be useful to have some knowledge of the overall system of accounting employed in the NHS or the independent sector.

Of these four topics the system for allocating resources and the accounting procedures in the NHS are the most complex and probably of least direct relevance to ward level managers. To understand the concepts of costing and budgets, however, it is necessary to place them in the context of this whole financial system.

FINANCING THE NHS

The annual resources used to provide a Health Service is in excess of £18 750 million (1986). Of this sum the greatest amount is obtained from Government National Exchequer with 86% of the total; 11% comes from National Insurance funds and 3% from other sources.

There are two main components of this fund. One is allocated to health authorities and the other is allocated to the Family Practitioner Committee (FPC) for GP services, dentists and opticians. (The method of fixing on the particular annual figure and the way this is allocated through the NHS structure to eventually meet the costs of health care across the country is complex.)

The first step is for Government to decide on a total level of public expenditure for a year. The next stage is to allocate proportions of this between the various public spending programmes (Education, Social Security, etc.). In advancing this process a Public Expenditure Survey Committee (PESC) has the task of identifying the appropriate priorities and reporting these to the Chancellor of the Exchequer. Next comes a White Paper on public expenditure which is a plan for spending, including assumptions on pay and price increases. After a debate on the context of the paper, funds are voted by Parliament through the authority of the Parliamentary Estimates Procedures.

In understanding the distribution of these finances within the NHS and FPC it is necessary to explain some basic concepts of public funding. First is the distinction between capital and revenue expenditures. Revenue refers to the money required for day-to-day running of the services (mostly wages and salaries). Capital is the money required for the acquisition of assets (new buildings, major equipment). A third category of expenditure is 'earmarked allocations' which refers to money for specific purposes which can be capital, or revenue, or both, and can either be funded entirely by a health authority, or jointly with a local authority.

Another important concept in NHS finance is that of 'cash limit'. Until 1976/77 the allocation of funds each year could be increased during the year to reflect the actual impact of inflation. This was arranged by means of a supplement voted by Parliament. Since 1977 the total allocation to the NHS has included a figure to cover the estimated rises in pay and prices. This remains fixed, irrespective of whether these costs are actually greater; thus a limit is imposed on the amount of cash DHAs can draw from the DHSS. The cash limit is not imposed on the FPC funds which thus remain open-ended to reflect the actual

demand for the service and the full increase in costs.

The cash limited figure for NHS expenditure has to be portioned out to the regional health authorities and thence to the DHAs. Here a further complication arises. The Health Service is intended to provide an equal resource in all communities but it has been estimated that the South East RHA contains more extensive facilities than the rest of the country. A formula has been devised, aimed at obtaining assessment of relative needs for health care in different parts of the country. This is referred to as the RAWP formula as it is a modification of proposals made by a Resources Allocation Working Party (1976). This calculation is complicated, but basically measures differences in population served by a RHA weighted by age, sex, and a standardised mortality ratio and adjusted for cross-boundary provisions. There are separate allowances to account for London weighting, teaching costs and provisions used by several regions.

The figure agreed is allocated by the DHSS to each RHA who in turn has the responsibility of allocating this between its DHAs, less the cost of regional services (HO, computers, blood transfusions) according to regional policy. In dividing the remainder, some regions use a RAWP approach; others make provision based on policy preferences for different services. Most regions hold funds for capital expenditure which are free of interest and do not have to be repaid. RHAs cannot borrow money, although they can promote fund-raising activities and dispose of unwanted capital assets. The DHAs draw cash from the DHSS each week to cover revenue expenditure.

HEALTH SERVICE ACCOUNTING

Each health authority has a statutory obligation not to exceed cash limits in requisitions to the DHSS. If this does happen, the overspending is liable to be carried over into the next year, thus reducing the sum available. Any underspending of allocation is lost except for 1% which can be carried forward; another option is to transfer from revenue to capital (1%) or capital to revenue (up to 10%).

Health authorities are also required to produce accounts for the DHSS which are audited both internally and externally by the National Audit office, to ensure proper financial controls have been applied.

It is useful for nurse managers to understand a little of the conventions that are used in producing accounts generally, and to appreciate how the Health Service modifies these for its particular circumstances. All businesses produce two documents which can be used to record their financial affairs over a specific period of time. One is a balance sheet: this shows the value of the undertaking at a particular time by indicating the funds invested which are termed 'liabilities' (capital employed, loans, creditors), and the 'assets' (buildings, equipment, stock, debtors and cash) which should be equal — hence the term balance sheet.

A distinction is drawn between 'fixed' assets which are those with an existence beyond the year of purchase (buildings. land, major equipment, etc.), and 'current' assets which are those to be used during the year (stocks, debtors, cash in bank, etc.).

The second financial record shows the state of income and expenditure which for businesses is termed the trading and profit and loss account. In business this report, which can be made for any period, but is usually produced annually, records the profitability of the company. This is the excess of income over expenditure in a trading period. There is a distinction between gross or trading profit and net profit. Gross profit is calculated by deducting the direct costs of manufacturing products or providing services (material used, direct labour costs, transport costs, etc.) from revenue obtained from the sale of the goods or services. These are the 'variable costs' in that they increase or fall in proportion to the quantity of business undertaken. Businesses also have a number of 'fixed costs' or 'overheads' which remain the same whatever the level of output (rates, rents, indirect labour costs, depreciation of fixed assets, etc.). When

this sum is deducted from the gross profit it gives the lower net profit (or net loss). This will be the profit before any taxes are paid. In seeking to control the finances of an undertaking in order to achieve its targets of a net profit or even break, business management is most concerned about 'cash flow'. This is the pattern of money being spent by a company compared with income earned.

Health authorities use most of these concepts in seeking to run their services in a cost-effective manner. They are required to prepare two sets of annual accounts. The income and expenditure account is drawn up using the normal conventions of a trading account except that there is no depreciation figure for capital assets. The balance sheet shows only the current assets (stock, debtors and cash) and the current liabilities (creditors); there is no statement about capital assets or liabilities. Each DHA is part of a financial system and is required to make additional accounting returns to the DHSS. One is a weekly requisition for cash required, together with a forecast of the requirement for the next three weeks. From December to March a copy of this return is sent to the appropriate RHA. If cash advance is likely to exceed cash limits the RHA is advised to take action. So Health Service managers are as concerned with 'cash flow' management as any business manager.

In trying to keep within a cash limit target they could reduce stock purchases to a minimum, defer payment of bills to the next financial year, and collect as much cash from debtors as possible. If this fails it may be possible to use reserve funds, transfer some capital to revenue expenditure, or finally reduce staff and services provided.

The acquisition of funds and the overall system of financial accounting in the NHS is far more complex than our generalised explanation, but for most nurse managers there is greater need to understand the concepts of costing and budgetary control as these are of direct relevance to managing efficiently and making appropriate decisions.

It is useful to consider these techniques in

general before looking at specific health care applications.

COST ACCOUNTING

In business and in the private health sector it is essential to be able to determine what are the actual costs of producing a commodity or providing a service so that this is taken into account in determining prices or giving bills to patients. In the public health sector this information is also of considerable benefit to managers in seeking to control costs, as expenditure responsibility can be identified, comparisons can be made with previous periods or pre-determined budgets, sources of waste can be pin-pointed and an analysis of total expenditure into 'fixed' and 'variable' costs can be made.

Cost accounting is concerned with sections of a business or organisation, both for provision of historic information on what a particular activity has cost, and to forecast what a future activity ought to cost. A 'cost' can be defined as the value of economic resources used as a result of producing or doing the thing costed. This consists of two components — quantity used and the price per unit. The thing that is costed is termed a 'cost unit' which can be units of production (syringes, surgical packs, cups of coffee, etc.) or units of service (inpatient day, outpatient client, etc.).

Costs can also be defined for parts of an organisation, called 'cost centres' (particular departments, wards, school health services etc.). Thus there are two stages in cost analysis. First is to allocate the appropriate expenses to various cost centres; second is to divide these costs between various cost units.

Costs are classified under two headings: 'Direct' (wages, materials, expenses) and 'indirect' (wages, materials, expenses). Direct wages means the cost of wages paid to staff immediately concerned with making a product or giving service to 'customers' (ward nursing staff, doctors, ambulance drivers, etc.). Direct materials means the cost of materials which become part of a product or service (drugs, bandages, etc.). Direct expenses means other costs that arise wholly from the existence of whatever is being costed (travel, fuel, etc.).

Indirect materials, wages and expenses covers all other expenditure, such as cleaning materials, stationery, payment for cleaners, supervisors, lighting, heating, etc. These indirect costs can also be considered as 'overheads', which in a business can be divided into production overheads, administration overheads, distribution overheads and selling overheads. These are calculated and apportioned to each cost centre to be included in producing total costs for each cost unit. There are several methods used for making this allocation.

Another useful way of analysing costs is to distinguish between 'fixed' and 'variable'. Fixed costs are those items not affected by the volume of output or level of service provided (rents, management salaries, some overheads, etc.). Variable costs are those items which fluctuate with changes in volume of output or service provided (direct labour, direct materials, etc.). A third category of cost is referred to as semi-variable or semi-fixed.

These concepts can be used by managers in commercial activities to identify a 'break even' point (the point where total costs per volume against the revenue from sales is equal).

There has been an increasing application of cost accounting both within the NHS and private health care.

Health authorities produce many cost statements which analyse the expenditure of each hospital and department on a functional basis, as the 'primary analysis', and expenditure on inpatients and outpatients, as well as breakdowns of costs per case, per inpatient day and per outpatient day. This data can be used to make comparisons between hospitals of the same type and can be used to establish standards of performance. There are further cost analyses for estate management, catering, radiography and the ambulance service. The community services are costed separately with analysis of school health service, general community care, preventive services and family planning.

BUDGETARY CONTROL

Budgetary control is found in most manufacturing and service industries as well as in the public services. Financial and cost accounting tends to concentrate on what has happened in the past and relate this to current activities. Budgets are a different form of financial control in that they are an expression in money (or sometimes quantitative) terms of what it is hoped will happen. Therefore budgets are part of planning and depend on forecasts about future demand. Once a budget has been established, it is a means of controlling expenditure if it provides a method of recording cost information. This enables a manager to monitor expenditures and decide if corrective action is needed.

In seeking a general understanding of budgetary control and its place in overall financial management it will be useful to clarify some further terminology.

Budget
: A financial or quantitative statement prepared and approved, prior to a defined period of time, or policy to be pursued during that period for the purpose of attaining given objectives

Variance
: The difference between the sum allowed in the budget and the actual amount spent: this variance is often expressed as a percentage of the budgeted amount

Budget Centre
: An area of responsibility in an organisation that is required to produce its own budget

Incremental budgeting
: The process whereby a budget is prepared based on previous periods with increased or decreased increments to allow for changes in activity level, inflation, service economies etc.

Zero-based budgeting
: The system of preparing a budget where every financial allocation has to be justified from first principles: each unit

and price included in the budget has to be justified from cost benefit considerations.

The overall budget for an RHA is an expression of how its revenue will be expended in a given period to meet its health care objectives. The overall plan is the master budget which is then subdivided between its hospital and other services from which departmental budgets are formed. If budgets are to be of practical benefit, they must be agreed between the budget holder and senior management rather than being imposed from above.

Within the NHS the basic information for budgeting must include budget holder, name of budget, period of time, target and spending. The budget can be calculated on the basis of patient week costs which are identified under three headings:

1. Overhead charge: heating, lights, rates, maintenance cleaning, etc.
2. Nursing and other salaries
3. Running expenses: drugs, provisions, laundry, etc.

The budget holder should receive a regular statement of expenditure as a budget period progresses. This will enable comparisons to be made with the planned expenditure. If there is a discrepancy, these are 'variances' which need to be accounted for and possibly corrective action taken to avoid overspending. The expenditures arising in a hospital budget can be distinguished between 'continuous predictable' (mainly payroll as it can be calculated and forecast), 'infrequent but predictable' (Bank holidays, sickness, study days, etc.), 'casual expenditure' (to meet a specific problem) and 'profiled expenditure' (heating, lighting costs follow a variable pattern over a budget period).

With information on expenditures provided regularly, the nurse manager as budget holder can calculate what remains for the rest of the budget period. It is unlikely that there will be exactly equal expenditure in this period (i.e. 50% of budget used as the half-way point), but budgetary control means that a manager must understand where her money is going and whether it will last until the end of the period.

NURSE MANAGERS AND FINANCE

During the 1980s there has been a greater emphasis within the NHS on financial control and constraint. The demand for health care has increased, the cost of providing high technology treatment has increased, the general pattern of inflation has meant that the cost of more traditional forms of nursing care has also increased.

Nurse managers as budget holders have a responsibility for helping the service achieve its 'value for money' objectives. They are involved in spending from their health authority's limited revenue budget. It is important that they ensure payment for staff is always correct, that supplies and stocks are used economically and are subject to proper monitoring. Nurse managers need to understand the 'standard financial instructions' issued by health authorities. They should be

a source of information on means of economising on unjustified expenditure, and should look for ways to improve the supply of stocks and services to a unit.

Some NHS staff are hostile to this 'business management' approach to running a caring service. This view ignores the reality of managing a public service which has to be financially accountable. Being financially aware and concerned is not incompatible with a caring and patient-centred attitude to nursing. The aim should be to ensure that no resources are wasted and that justifications for increases need to take into account the cost implications.

REFERENCES

Bryans W 1985 Money matters and other articles. In Nursing Times, March 13th, April 7th, and May 8th
Jones T, Prowle M 1982 Health service finance, Certified accountants Educational Trust, London
Lister A, Webber C 1985 Patient costing exercise, Nursing Times, February
Long A, Harrison S 1985 Health service performance, Croom Helm, London
Moss D 1984 Managing finance, In: Rowden R (ed) Managing nursing. Bailliere Tindall, London

Applications to health care

Computer basics

Managing with computers

23
Computers and nurse managers

In running management training programmes for a number of different organisations, I often ask managers to specify one feature of their organisation they would like to see improved. A frequent answer is 'A computer system that actually works.'

This illustrates one of the problems in the application of computers to business and public services. The aim should be to improve management control, to aid decision-making, and to improve the quality of service and products provided. To achieve this the line managers and non-computer specialists need to be involved in the specification of what they need from a computer system rather than let computer experts introduce systems they believe will benefit the organisation.

Health care has benefited from the application of computer technology and has potential for further beneficial uses. All nurse managers need to appreciate this potential and to be influential in trying to ensure that the applications are used for the benefit of patient care and the efficient operation of a health service. Nurse managers should therefore have a broad appreciation of what computers can do and how they do it.

APPLICATIONS TO HEALTH CARE

Computers can carry out arithmetic, manipulative and processing operations on 'business' data. The computer is a collection of electronic devices which has to be controlled by means of a program of instructions. The term 'hardware' is used to describe all the tangible pieces of a computer; 'software' describes the programs of instructions.

Within health care the need to process data and carry out arithmetic and manipulative activities with information is widespread. Computers have been used to speed up and extend the scope of these tasks within a health service for over twenty years. These applications can be classified as:

— Administration (finance, supply and statistics, etc)
— Hospital and primary care (patient admissions, appointments, medical records, etc)
— Scientific and clinical systems (laboratories, electro-cardiographic departments, etc)
— Management information systems (budgetary control, stock control, etc).

Line managers in nursing services will be affected by each of these types of application. They will have to supply data for input into health authority administration systems; they should be able to make use of systems giving information about patient admissions, records and so on; they should receive information through management systems which give greater ability to control a unit by understanding, with great speed and accuracy, variations from budget and use of supplies, as well as in planning rotas and treatments.

As there is an increasing amount of specific training on computer application and keyboard skills for health care managers and staff, as well as a considerable number of introductory books on computers, we include only a basic introduction to the topic in this chapter.

COMPUTER BASICS

There are five conceptual components in all computers: input, output, storage, arithmetic and logic, control.

The way data within the computer is represented and manipulated is based fundamentally on binary arithmetic. This is of little significance to a manager but it will be useful to appreciate the jargon terms 'a bit', 'a byte', and 'a word'.

This numbering system is designed using the base 2; each digit can only take the value of 0 or 1 (5 is 101 and 13 is 1011). There are two digits or 'bits'. A user is mainly concerned with the power and capacity of a computer which is expressed as x thousand bytes or words of storage. A byte is 8 bits; a word contains 16 or 24 bits, depending on the manufacturer. With 8 bits it is possible to represent any decimal digit, any letter of the alphabet and any range of special characters.

Data and instructions are entered into a computer in a variety of ways — punched cards, punched paper tape, magnetic tapes or disks, equipment to read characters optically or magnetically, keyboards and light pens. In future, handwritten and voice input facilities are likely to be developed.

The means by which computers communicate the results of data processes (output) are by line or character printers or by visual display units (VDUs) consisting of a keyboard and screen similar to a television set.

There are two basic types of storage associated with computers — working storage and backing storage. The working store is the main memory which contains the program(s) to carry out processing and control activities, which compiles information for output and in which all calculations, data manipulations and processing takes place. The size is an important measure of a computer's capacity which is expressed in thousands of bytes (32Kb memory) and indicates the size of file records which can be manipulated, the complexity of programs to be carried out and number of terminals that can be connected.

The backing store extends the capacity of a computer memory with data stored on magnetic tape or magnetic disks. There are two jargon terms associated with computer memory, ROM meaning 'read only memory' containing instructions to the computer, and RAM meaning 'random access memory' which can be controlled by the user.

Computers perform fundamentally simple arithmetic and logic functions — addition, subtraction, multiplication, division and comparison — but at very high speeds. The control unit of the computer is the 'brain' which selects program instructions from the working storage, interprets them, and activates input, storage, arithmetic, logic and output devices.

All this activity within a computer is activated and controlled by programs (software) which are lists of instructions (read, write, add, etc.) which have been compiled by a programmer based on an assessment of need made by a systems analyst to complete a particular job (district payroll, hospital appointments, etc). The instructions have to be expressed in a form that the control unit of a particular computer will understand. 'High level' language has been developed for this purpose — COBOL (Common Business Oriented Language), RPG (Report Program Generator language), Fortran (Formula translation), PLI and Basic. These are procedural languages and have disadvantages, and these have led to efforts to develop 'Fourth Generation languages' designed to facilitate the production of computer application programs. These are more 'user friendly' which can be used by non-professionals through micro-computers.

The problems in computer systems in not completing the tasks required are generally the result of program failures. Thus, selection of existing programs or development of a special program is of fundamental importance to managers who will be users of an application. Broadly, there are three types of software. Firstly, 'systems software' is supplied for a particular computer, giving programming languages an operating system and programs to control interface with terminals, communication facilities, etc. Then there is 'utilities software', which includes programs to carry out functions common to much of the computer processing carried out by users (sorting–merging data, dumping or copying data, generation of printed reports, etc.). Finally, 'applications software' is specific to particular problems which a user requires the computer to solve. As there are many common problems, applications software has been developed and sold to users for tasks such as payroll, stock control, financial management, personnel records, etc. The alternative is to write programs for a particular task, but this often requires many 'man years' of work and therefore considerable cost. As costs of hardware have fallen and the power of micro-and mini-computers has increased, there is considerable emphasis on selecting hardware because of the available software facilities.

There are three different ways in which computers process information. 'Batching processing' was the original and is still the most common (weekly and monthly payroll), where data is collected, coded, prepared for input and processed on a regular, predetermined basis. There will be manual computer interaction by input preparation, file handling, output control, but in between processing there is no updating of computer files and thus they are not a reflection of the real position. 'Real time processing' enables inputs to immediately update a record and this is a reflection of an actual circumstance. For applications such as hospital appointments, or bed allocations there is a need for up-to-date knowledge of available beds, immediate recording of a reservation and a barrier on allocating reserved beds for the next transaction.

'On line processing' gives the facility of access to enter for updating and enquiry. A real time system must be on line but on line need not operate in real time.

It is possible to make a broad distinction between three types of computing power — micro-computers, mini-computers and main frame computers. The micro has become familiar to many people through the development of 'home' computers. They are cheap; the central device, consisting of the logic, control circuitry, memory, a keyboard and a screen, can be acquired for a few hundred pounds. There are limitations in internal speed, in the size of the backing store and speed of printing. There is a large range of systems software supplied with machines and an increasing amount of application packages available and technical development which is overcoming some of the limitations.

The mini-computers overlap with micros at the bottom end of their range and with main frames at the other. They are faster, have a more comprehensive repertoire for programming, have larger storage, can support a network of terminals and can communicate with other computers.

The largest 'main frame' computers are capable of processing instructions in millions per second, with backing storage for thousands of millions of characters. They can have multiple input–outputs, can support large terminal networks and run several jobs at once. At this level, computing requires professional data processing staff.

Many organisations have recognised the benefit of computing, but rather than purchase their own equipment have used the facilities offered by a specialist 'computer bureau'. With the NHS during the 1970s regional computer bureau facilities were developed to support financial, statistical and other administrative services to districts using standardised main frame machines. These also provided terminals or mini-computer links in hospitals to deal with patient administration and hospital organisation.

MANAGING WITH COMPUTERS

Much of the application of computers in the NHS over the past twenty years has been directed towards administration tasks (process payroll, accounts, hospital activity analysis, etc.) or in support of work in pathological laboratories. Here we are concerned with the use of computers for management problems, particularly for the delivery of care services in hospitals or in the community. It is necessary for nurse managers to have some awareness of the possible benefits to managers in planning, control and decision-making, and for more senior nurse managers to be able to

influence Health Service management, so that the benefits of computer application should be directed at improving the practice of patient care.

Planning, whether long term and strategic, medium term and tactical or short-term operational, requires managers to process information. Information may be provided by manual processes or by computer systems, or both. Where, as in the case of NHS, an organisation already uses computers for administration and operational procedures, it can be possible to produce analyses or summaries of current and historic data held within existing systems for use in planning. There are also possibilities of using software packages of planning models which enable managers to ask 'What if . . . . .?' questions in trying to evaluate various courses of action. Microcomputer software is increasingly able to offer this type of help, especially with the development of 'spreadsheet' software. This makes it possible to compare the admission, treatment, length of stay, discharge and nature of each case for all consultants from a display on a VDU. It is possible to compare bed occupancy and study patient movements in a similar manner.

Computer systems can be applied to the process of planning and control, administration and supply requirements of patient services with such tasks as admitting and progressing patients, scheduling of outpatient appointments and maintenance of waiting lists. The five part forms used in some hospitals to administer a patient can be replaced by entry into a computer file which stores the required information and initiates the necessary administrative activities.

The planning process incorporates that of control if there is reliable feedback of information to management. Computers should be beneficial here if information is processed which gives a reliable indication of the level of service which is available with existing resources. There are other advantages in a reduction of time spent on administration tasks and an increase in the ability of hospital staff to be flexible in response to community demands with fast access to updated information.

It is clear that effective management depends on information that is useful, reliable and available at the appropriate time. In theory, computers have much to offer in the development of information systems. There is evidence, however, that they either provide similar information to that of previous manual systems or information that a computer professional believes user managers need. Line managers and specialist management staff should try to make the most use of information which is available but should also be encouraged to have greater influence in the selection of software or the development of internal computer systems. The proper definition in the design of systems will enable many routine decisions to be automated.

For such developments to be of real benefit to operational managers it is necessary to have on-line updating instead of batch processing, and on-line enquiry facilities to supplement fixed internal reporting and relevant information available in the computer. The advance of micro-computing and the 'database' approach should facilitate this.

The original approach to computer applications in organisations produced specific 'files' of information for each job the computer tackled. This means duplication of data — employee details may be repeated in payroll, personnel information and pensions applications. These files are updated at different times and amendments to records can have an impact on many programs. Thus there has been a development of the database approach, which means having a single computer file for a whole organisation, or at least separate databases serving a group of related applications. There is an increasing amount of database software available for all levels of computing including micros.

There are immense problems for existing computer users with conventional data processing file structures in converting to database. Within health care it is likely that new local applications using small computers will adopt this approach, while larger existing applications will be modified gradually.

As users of management information it is useful for senior nurses to review their need for information in carrying out their own jobs. What are the key decisions that you have to make? What information do you need to make these decisions? How useful is the information provided by manual and computer systems now? When is information needed? Is any information provided too soon or too late?

Such a review will enable a nurse manager to make full use of information already available through a hospital or district system, to request changes in the times when some is delivered, to ignore some identified as irrelevant and to make constructive requests for improvement when a computerised system is introduced or modified.

Managing people and managing information are the essential skills for effective managers. It is certain that health care, like all other organisations, will be subject to more extensive computerisation in future and therefore that all nurse managers and ambitious nurses will need to equip themselves with a deeper appreciation of the topics that have been introduced in this chapter, as well as getting to grips with the practical skills needed to use the computer equipment and systems that are becoming increasingly available to health care managers.

REFERENCES

Collen M 1974 Hospital computer systems, John Wiley & Son, Chichester
Cowen P 1983 Managing with computers. Pan, London
Punnell B K, Jackson D C, Lucas S B 1986 Introducing microcomputers. Hodder and Stoughton Teach Yourself Books, Sevenoaks

Index